SpringerBriefs in Public Health present concise summaries of cutting-edge research and practical applications from across the entire field of public health, with contributions from medicine, bioethics, health economics, public policy, biostatistics, and sociology.

The focus of the series is to highlight current topics in public health of interest to a global audience, including health care policy; social determinants of health; health issues in developing countries; new research methods; chronic and infectious disease epidemics; and innovative health interventions.

Featuring compact volumes of 50 to 125 pages, the series covers a range of content from professional to academic. Possible volumes in the series may consist of timely reports of state-of-the art analytical techniques, reports from the field, snapshots of hot and/or emerging topics, elaborated theses, literature reviews, and in-depth case studies. Both solicited and unsolicited manuscripts are considered for publication in this series.

Briefs are published as part of Springer's eBook collection, with millions of users worldwide. In addition, Briefs are available for individual print and electronic purchase.

Briefs are characterized by fast, global electronic dissemination, standard publishing contracts, easy-to-use manuscript preparation and formatting guidelines, and expedited production schedules. We aim for publication 8–12 weeks after acceptance.

More information about this series at https://link.springer.com/bookseries/10138

Fábio Silveira
Arlene Terezinha Cagol Garcia Badoch

Effective Public Health Policy in Organ Donation

Lessons from a Universal Public
Health System in Brazil

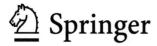 Springer

Fábio Silveira (iD)
Centro Digestivo e Transplante de
Órgãos - CDTO
Hospital do Rocio
Campo Largo, Paraná, Brazil

Arlene Terezinha Cagol Garcia Badoch
Central Estadual de Transplantes do Paraná
Curitiba, Paraná, Brazil

ISSN 2192-3698   ISSN 2192-3701   (electronic)
SpringerBriefs in Public Health
ISBN 978-3-030-99287-3   ISBN 978-3-030-99288-0   (eBook)
https://doi.org/10.1007/978-3-030-99288-0

This Springer imprint is published by the registered company Springer Nature Switzerland AG
The registered company address is: Gewerbestrasse 11, 6330 Cham, Switzerland

Contents

Chapter 1
The Paraná Model of Organ Donation and Transplant

An Overview of the Brazilian Health and Transplant System

Brazil manages and runs the world's major public transplant program. The transplant medicine evolution required an adaptation and modernization of the overall framework from the public authorities and professional organizations, which was imperative for operating such a complex system.

The Brazilian transplant system is part of the National Health System (SUS), a universal access system established by the 1988 Constitution as an outcome of the Brazilian society transition from an authoritarian regimen to a democratic one(Vasconcelos & Pasche, 2012).

Brazil is a presidential republican federative system composed of 27 states and one federal district, where the country's capital is. The states are composed of municipalities. Therefore, the SUS system connects these three levels of government health organizations (municipalities, states, and federal government), and it's not limited to assistance services.

SUS constitutional basis is universality, integrality, and equity, following the decentralization, regionalization, hierarchization, and community participation guidelines. Comparatively, SUS is not a market system such as the North American or welfare such as in France and Germany. It's similar to the national public systems of the United Kingdom, Canada, Spain, and Portugal.

The description of the SUS organization is relevant because it highlights how Paraná State Transplant System – as described in this writing – improved over the past decade based on the actions of the state managers, a not even development in other Brazilian states, although they are submitted to the same legal framework.

The legal characteristics of the Brazilian transplant system began to evolve in the late 1950s and are currently grounded on the prohibition of organ and tissue trade, donation after brain death diagnosis principles, and only upon family authorization.

© The Author(s), under exclusive license to Springer Nature Switzerland AG 2022
F. Silveira, A. T. C. G. Badoch, *Effective Public Health Policy in Organ Donation*,
SpringerBriefs in Public Health, https://doi.org/10.1007/978-3-030-99288-0_1

The transplant waiting lists are statewide. Non-heart-beating donor modality is not regulated in Brazil.

Despite its universal nature, SUS faces the shortcomings of a developing country, chronically underfinanced. Brazil stands in the 84th Human Development Index (HDI 0.765) world ranking (PNUD, 2020), and its funding is criticized as the resource distribution has been mainly determined by federal agents, the disadvantage of the states, and municipalities' autonomy.

Paraná State is situated in the southern region of Brazil and has a gross revenue per capita higher than the national. In addition, we must acknowledge that despite the difficulties, the transplant system could not have developed amid a poorly structured health system. To be part of SUS and Paraná State's reality was crucial to building the history described in this writing. Paraná State's Transplant Center was one of Brazil's pioneers, founded in 1995 by a state ordinance, which constituted the Special Group for Organs and Tissues Transplantation. This work established the regulatory basis for the state's activity and provided support to the national legislation, which set up the National Transplant System (Borges, 2014).

From 2011 to 2020, actions adopted by the Paraná State Transplant Center sought to improve the state's transplant system. Despite previously presenting brain death detection and effective donation activity, the state's numbers were below those expected for the state's socioeconomic development level compared to the Brazilian reality.

The Donation As a Consequence of Brain Death Identification

Physicians make clinical decisions several times throughout their work. They are prepared to collect data through anamnesis, physical examination, and complementary exam analysis. The consequence is the establishment of a potential diagnosis or differential diagnosis.

The permanent cease of any activity of the central nervous system is a clinical condition that characterizes brain death; its recognition is a medical diagnosis.

Severe brain damage leads to the interruption of all cerebral blood flow; although breathing is maintained through artificial means as the heart maintains its rhythm, it is an entity undeniably accepted as death. The steps and methods to this diagnostic confirmation are well established and determined by the Medicine Federal Council regulation (Medicina, 2017).

The brain-dead patient is considered a potential organ donor. To picture the brain death diagnosis merely as a means of obtaining organs and tissues for transplant is fundamentally untrue. It is a diagnosis that, besides technical, as human (Medicina, 2019), is a legal right, as the family must know if its relative is either dead or alive.

This is how the transplant journey begins, with a diagnosis establishment. The brain death diagnosis, although mandatory and of compulsory notification, was not a reality in Paraná State. Therefore, the most important step of the transplant system readjustment was that **the culture of brain death diagnosis should be fostered**.

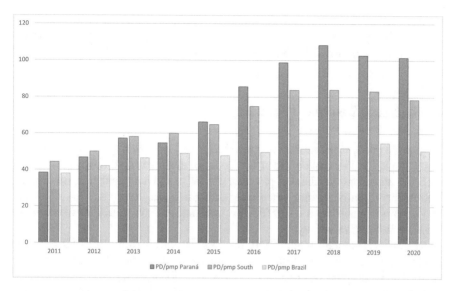

Fig. 1.1 Relative growth of potential donors' numbers in Paraná, southern region, and Brazil. (*pmp* per million population, *PD* potential donor)

Table 1.1 Number of potential donors identified in Paraná, southern region, and Brazil

Year	PD/pmp PR	PD/pmp South	PD/pmp BR
2011	38.4	44.3	37.9
2012	46.7	50	42.1
2013	57.2	58.1	46.5
2014	54.6	60	49
2015	66.2	64.8	47.8
2016	85.6	74.9	49.7
2017	98.8	83.8	51.6
2018	108.3	84	51.9
2019	102.7	83.2	54.7
2020	101.5	78.5	50.5

pmp per million population, *PR* Paraná State, *South* southern region, *BR* Brazil

In the last decade, the Paraná State has gradually increased the detection of potential donors, surpassing the rate of 100 potential donors per million population. This growth did not happen with only the state itself as a reference but also in regard to Brazil (+36.61%) and the country's southern region (+10.31%) – the one with the most similar socioeconomic development (Fig. 1.1 and Table 1.1).

The brain death identification is performed through an active search system, where the team of Intra-Hospital Committee on Organ and Tissue Donation for Transplants (CIHDOTT) alongside the Organ Procurement Organization (OPO) works within the critical hospital units monitoring cases that could potentially lead to the diagnosis.

The CIHDOTT role is not to determine the diagnosis – this is a medical action – but rather to provide the necessary conditions for the diagnostic process. **The donation is a consequence of the brain death diagnosis**.

Beforehand, Disregard Metrics

Targets are good, set goals, and organize processes. However, the setting of a diagnostic target for potential donors at first does not make sense. And why?

Estimates on the numbers of potential donors in a given population are diverse. Ratio per million population (PMP), regarding hospital death numbers, of deaths that happen in intensive care unit (ICU) is used, and all have something in common, the large forecast variability.

Regarding potential donors/PMP, the forecast varies from 30 to 60 per year (Goldberg et al., 2017; Matesanz & Dominguez-Gil, 2007; ONT, 1999; Sheehy et al., 2003), hospital deaths from 1 to 4% (Goldberg et al., 2017; Matesanz & Dominguez-Gil, 2007), and deaths in the ICU of 10–40% (Garcia, 2000; Gore et al., 1992). As it is observed, there is an inherent difficulty in setting goals based on such stretched range objectives.

This width is due to different demographic patterns, hospital care networks, and the investigation of the different populations' health systems.

Paraná overcame this estimate difficulty with the implementation of a slightly clearer target: **identify all brain deaths**. This motto fosters the culture of brain death diagnosis, draws away from the focus number in potential, mobilizes the teams to pursue excellence, and strengthens the perception that donation is a consequence of this process.

Understanding the Organization Format

The State Transplant Center is an entity linked to the Paraná State Health Secretariat, which is subordinated to the National Transplant System. Following the decentralized nature of the National Health System (SUS), each state is responsible for managing its system. This administrative autonomy results in the different organ donation rates found across our federation states.

Despite being independent, their responsibilities and duties were defined by federal normative acts – Ordinance 2600/2009 (BRASIL, 2009) – later replaced by the Consolidation Ordinance no. 04/2017 (BRASIL, 2017). The National Transplant System's General Coordination, advised by a Strategic Counselling Group, encompassed by different hues involved in the process, is the federal government body that oversees the State Transplant Centers, coordinates the distribution of organs across the states, and updates current standards and guidelines.

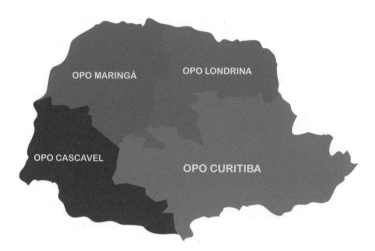

Fig. 1.2 OPOs' arrangement in Paraná State

Paraná State Transplant Center, following the decentralization logic, established the Organ Procurement Organizations (OPO), namely, OPO Curitiba, OPO Maringá, OPO Londrina, and OPO Cascavel (Fig. 1.2). These OPOs are responsible for the municipalities that are part of the health regional offices in their field of expertise.

The regional health offices that comprise the OPOs are listed in Table 1.2.

OPOs are not private organizations. They are linked to the State Central, composed of stated career professionals. **The governmental nature of all OPOs is unique in State Transplant Centers across the country**.

CIHDOTTs are mandatory in public, private, and philanthropic hospitals that fit into profiles related to the number of deaths and sort of available beds, according to ordinance 2600 and its following consolidation (BRASIL, 2017). They are the institution's responsibility, and its members are nursing professionals and/or physicians. The number of CIHDOTTS grew at first; afterward, it did not vary widely from year to year, as it mirrors the existing hospital structure (Fig. 1.3).

This organizational design was in effect at the beginning of 2011, however with a delivery of results for the population below the desired (Dell Agnolo et al., 2012) due to Paraná State level of human development (Silveira, 2011).

The country's fifth economy, of recognized social strength, bitterly ranked the eighth position in the national donation ranking, with an 8.7 rate of effective donors/ PMP (ABTO, 2010).

In an early diagnosis, both state coordination and OPOs lacked organizational flows, standard operating procedures, and professionals with *expertise* in the different process stages. **It was necessary to change this**.

The combined action of the OPOs and the CIHDOTTs within hospital institutions, under the supervision of the State Central, should constitute the active search system, and this system was gradually improved, with the establishment of the "Paraná State Transplant Excellence Program" (CIB/PR, 2013).

Table 1.2 The regional health offices that comprise the OPOs

Regional Health Office	OPO
1ª RS- Paranaguá	
2ª RS- Curitiba	
3ª RS- Ponta Grossa	Curitiba
4ª RS- Irati	
5ª RS- Guarapuava	
6ª RS- União da Vitória	
7ª RS- Pato Branco	
8ª RS- Francisco Beltrão	Cascavel
9ª RS- Foz do Iguaçu	
10ª RS- Cascavel	
11ª RS- Campo Mourão	
12ª RS- Umuarama	
13ª RS- Cianorte	Maringá
14ª RS- Paranavaí	
15ª RS- Maringá	
16ª RS- Apucarana	
17ª RS- Londrina	
18ª RS- Cornélio Procópio	Londrina
19ª RS- Jacarezinho	
20ª RS- Toledo	Cascavel
21ª RS- Telêmaco Borba	Curitiba
22ª RS- Ivaiporã	Londrina

The decentralized nature of the system, in pursuit of operational autonomy for the OPOs, was designed as an effective template for increasing the potential donors' base (Fig. 1.4). Despite seeking the improvement of the largest centers, most of the donations take place in the smaller centers, which are not prepared for transplants.

This decentralization and stimulation of the brain death diagnosis culture, performed in intensive care settings, can be found in Fig. 1.5, which demonstrates a progressive increase (+34%) of the notifying hospitals' numbers, mostly in hospitals without established transplant services.

While tracing the number of potential donors annually identified in the five largest reporting centers in the last decade, we observe that they were responsible for 28.17% of the donations (Fig. 1.6).

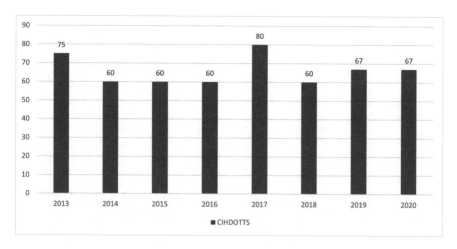

Fig. 1.3 Number of CIHDOTTs established each year

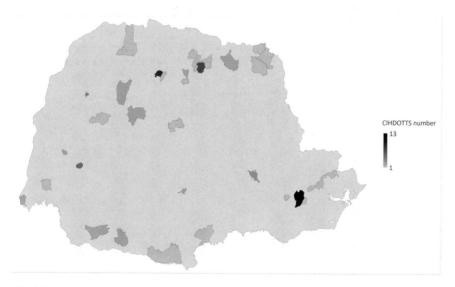

Fig. 1.4 Municipalities with active CIHDOTTs

Attempting to maximize the notification and donation effectiveness process in a few centers of expertise can be tempting to the manager as, theoretically, it increases the control of the involved variables. However, this was not the desired outcome, **it was necessary to move the system out of its comfort zone**, and the wager was to develop the brain death diagnosis culture in as many hospitals as possible.

When expanding the analysis to the top ten notifying centers, it is noticeable that an average of 49.48% of the total potential donors was identified there. Over the last years of the decade, it's possible to see that about 55% up to 60% of potential donors were identified outside the ten largest centers (Fig. 1.7).

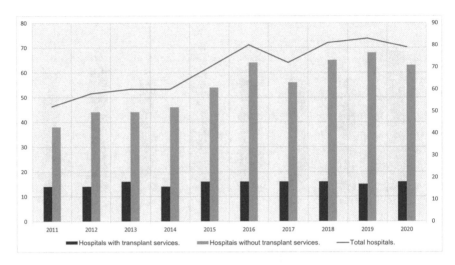

Fig. 1.5 Number of hospitals with notification of potential donors

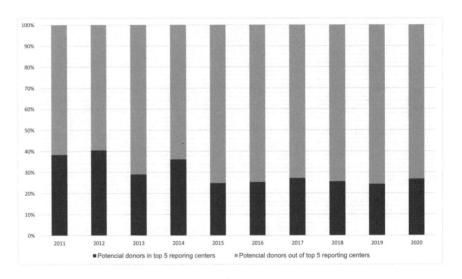

Fig. 1.6 Frequency of potential donors identified in the five largest reporting centers

This data shows the relevance of the system's expansiveness reach, several centers with effective search activity. In this decade, the centers that is most frequently featured in the first positions were Cajuru University Hospital and Rocio Hospital, based in Curitiba and Campo Largo, respectively.

In a theoretical scenario of exclusive notification within the ten largest centers of the decade, the average of potential donors/PMP would be 38.47, below the national average of 48.17 potential donors/PMP in the same period.

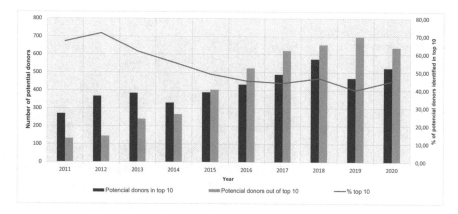

Fig. 1.7 Potential donors identified in the ten largest reporting centers

The State Transplant System has built its development base by following the SUS decentralization and regionalization organizational principle.

The System's Inspiration

The method of intrahospital operation to actively seek potential donors is based on the Spanish design considered the gold standard of the organizational systems of organ procurement and distribution in the world.

This rearranged model from the late 1980s is based on the "transplant coordinator" role in the hospital (Matesanz et al., 2017), being responsible for the local search. This coordinator, majorly intensive care physicians, works together with nursing assistance, under direct subordination to the hospitals' medical director.

The Spanish main office, the National Organization of Transplants (ONT), has a supporting agency nature. Its quality system is based on medical record review, internal and external audits, and coordination of autonomous communities, our State Transplant Centers' equivalent. ONT has no specific executive competence.

In addition to active search activities, the Spanish hospital coordination seeks to emphasize training, whether of coordinators, ICU doctors and nurses, and emergency departments.

The Brazilian system is based on the Spanish system but is not identical to it. This template proposed by the Brazilian Organ Transplant Association (Garcia, 2000) was nationally adopted (Fig. 1.8). In it, the federation states have regulatory, distribution, and inspection roles and hold organizational autonomy. This autonomy led Paraná to implement some modifications, aiming for the system's improvement and its adjustment to the local reality.

Both Spain and Brazil have public health systems based on universal access, a feature that contributes to the efficiency of a transplant system (Matesanz, 2001).

Fig. 1.8 Organizational
comparison of the Spanish
and Brazilian transplant
systems

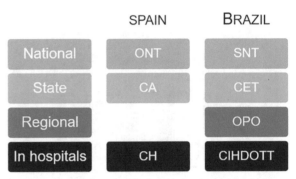

ONT – National Organization of Transplants; **SNT** – National Transplant
System; **CA** – Autonomic Communities; **CET** – State Transplant Center;
OPO – Organ Procurement Organization; **CH** – Hospital Coordination;
CIHDOTT – Intra-Hospital Organ and Tissue Donation Commission for
Transplantation.

In Spain, autonomous coordination has an audit and quality control nature; it's not assigned as an intrahospital activity. Paraná equivalent, the CET, encourages the OPOs to seek out hospitals, to work in loco together with the CIHDOTTs.

The Spanish hospital coordination, engaged in overcoming the obstacles of the family approach and identification of potential donors (Matesanz et al., 1994), has its attributions levelled by the CIHDOTT in the Brazilian system.

This is an activity that does not follow business hours; therefore, encouraging OPO's presence in notifying hospitals contributes to the solution of issues that are most frequent in smaller hospitals and that don't have the appropriate capacity to handle all the stages of the process. The personnel and financial structures of CIHDOTTs are mainly weaker than those of OPOs.

National legislation does not require CIHDOTT staff members' full-time availability. Nevertheless, a Paraná-wide regulation was established requiring that all transplant centers must have intrahospital commission staff, working on an exclusive dedication regime.

The reasoning behind this determination is that responsible transplant centers should set an example for other hospitals.

Thus, the unique organizational characteristics of the Paraná system is threefold:

1. Unlike Brazilian peers, all OPOs are state-owned.
2. Unlike the Brazilian model, OPOs need to work within notifying hospitals.
3. Unlike the Spanish model, CIHDOTTs do not necessarily rely on physicians

These differences **classify the Paraná system as a hybrid**, a modification of the Spanish and Brazilian versions.

How Active Search and Diagnostic Confirmation Work

Patients with severe brain damage, in a coma that does not respond to stimulation, and in need of breathing support through mechanical ventilation are possible donors. The most common causes of these situations are vascular accidents and trauma. These patients under mechanical ventilation have physical examination signs, combined with the inability to maintain spontaneous ventilation, which is identified in the daily care rounds in intensive care units (Tannous et al., 2018).

It is a responsibility of the CIHDOTT's team to visit the ICUs on a daily basis and evaluate patients who have these suggestive clinical conditions of brain death. In case of brain death suspicion, along with the ICU team, a diagnostic process is initiated, at which point the OPO must be notified. In this decade, an increase in the total number of potential donor notifications has been noticed in all OPOs in the state (Fig. 1.9 and Table 1.3).

The suspected diagnosis must be reported to the patient's family (República, 2017) by the ICU medical staff (Medicina, 2017). At this stage, the patient is considered a potential donor. Until the diagnosis is confirmed and the family has understood the diagnosis, **under no circumstances an approach regarding donations should be made**.

Clinical issues concerning the patient may prevent him from being an organ donor. At this stage of the process of the brain death identification, any potential formal or relative counterindication for donation **must not be considered**. As emphasized previously, the brain death diagnosis is a patient's and family's right, regardless of the potential for organ donation or not.

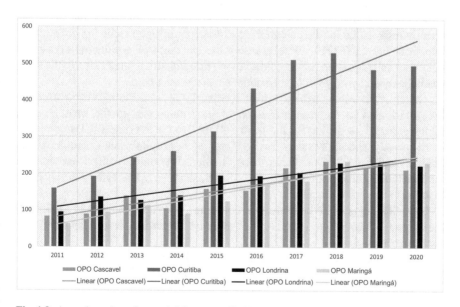

Fig. 1.9 Annual number of potential donors notified by OPOs

Table 1.3 Potential donor protocols opened according notifying OPO

	2011	2012	2013	2014	2015	2016	2017	2018	2019	2020	Total
OPO Cascavel	83	89	139	105	158	154	216	234	218	212	1608
OPO Curitiba	160	192	244	261	315	433	511	530	485	496	3627
OPO Londrina	95	136	127	140	195	194	203	230	230	223	1773
OPO Maringá	63	94	113	91	125	175	180	234	233	231	1539

Diagnostic confirmation requires several physical examination routine with regular intervals, diagnostic tests, and imaging examinations confirmations (Medicina, 2017). The CIHDOTT does not perform the exams; nevertheless, it works as an aid to the unit physician to confirm timetables, schedule exams, fill out legal forms, and contact the patient's family. **It is an enabler of the effective process for the ICU staff**.

The National Health System (SUS) is composed of hospitals with different technological capabilities for diagnosing brain death. While part of the protocol is performed at the bedside, its confirmation needs additional exams, whether it is the electroencephalogram, cerebral angiography, scintigraphy, or transcranial Doppler. **One of the weaknesses of a donation system is the inability to perform these tests**. This issue was mapped in the state, according to the particularity of each OPO, and solutions were deployed, enabling, through cooperation agreements or direct funding, the possibility to conduct diagnostic tests within the SUS.

Therefore, the nonmandatory presence of a physician in the CIHDOTTs is counterbalanced through the presence, at the State Transplant Center, of available physicians with degrees and intensive care experience, on a daily basis, as technical support to the physicians of the notifying hospitals.

This sort of support is triggered not only under the request of the physician directly responsible for the potential organ donor care. Upon receiving the notification from the CIHDOTT/OPO regarding the existence of a potential donor, the CET's on-call physician gets in contact to provide support, related either to the brain death diagnostic process or to the patient's maintenance care.

Therefore, focusing on the physician specialist role in the State Transplant Center has contributed to the standardization of procedures and to the system's cost improvement. This distinction has been well received in the state's ICUs.

Eventually, potential donors can be identified in hospitals that do not have formally established CIHDOTTs. In these situations, the on-duty physician contacts the local OPO, which, followed by the contact, sends over the team to the hospital, to assist in the entire process.

Once the diagnosis of brain death is confirmed, the patient's death is confirmed; the diagnosis must be explained to the family by the medical team responsible for the treatment.

The diagnostic record of brain death is a quality tool for the ICU, the hospital, and the healthcare system itself (Duarte, 2019; Gois et al., 2017).

References

ABTO. (2010). In V. D. Garcia (Ed.), *RBT - Registro Brasileiro de Transplantes*. ABTO - Associação Brasileira de Transplante de Órgãos.

Borges, H. F. (2014). In H. D. F. Borges (Ed.), *Manual de Transplantes* (3rd ed.). Central Estadual de Transplantes do Paraná.

BRASIL. (2009). In M. D. Saúde (Ed.), *Portaria n°2600, de 21 de outubro de 2009*. Diário Oficial da União.

BRASIL. (2017). *Portaria de Consolidação n°4, de 28 de setembro de 2017*. Ministério da Saúde.

CIB/PR. (2013). In C. D. S. M. D. S. D. Paraná & S. D. E. D. S. D. Paraná (Eds.), *Comissão intergestores bipartite do Paraná - Deliberação n°377*. Conselho de Secretários Municipais de Saúde do Paraná.

Dell Agnolo, C. M., De Freitas, R. A., Toffolo, V. J., De Oliveira, M. L., De Almeida, D. F., Carvalho, M. D., & Pelloso, S. M. (2012). Causes of organ donation failure in Brazil. *Transplantation Proceedings, 44*, 2280–2282.

Duarte, G. F. (2019). *Construção de processo avaliativo para comissões intra-hospitalares de transplante*. Universidade Estadual de Maringá.

Garcia, V. D. (2000). *Por uma política de transplantes no Brasil*. São Paulo.

Gois, R., Galdino, M., Pissinati, P., Pimentel, R., Carvalho, M., & Haddad, M. (2017). Efetividade do processo de doação de órgãos para transplantes. *Acta Paulista de Enfermagem [online], 30*, 621–627.

Goldberg, D., Kallan, M. J., Fu, L., Ciccarone, M., Ramirez, J., Rosenberg, P., Arnold, J., Segal, G., Moritsugu, K. P., Nathan, H., Hasz, R., & Abt, P. L. (2017). Changing metrics of organ procurement organization performance in order to increase organ donation rates in the United States. *American Journal of Transplantation, 17*, 3183–3192.

Gore, S. M., Cable, D. J., & Holland, A. J. (1992). Organ donation from intensive care units in England and Wales: Two year confidential audit of deaths in intensive care. *BMJ, 304*, 349–355.

Matesanz, R. (2001). Transplantations, management, and health systems. *Nefrologia, 21*(Suppl 4), 3–12.

Matesanz, R., & Dominguez-Gil, B. (2007). Strategies to optimize deceased organ donation. *Transplantation Reviews, 21*, 177–188.

Matesanz, R., Dominguez-Gil, B., Coll, E., Mahillo, B., & Marazuela, R. (2017). How Spain reached 40 deceased organ donors per million population. *American Journal of Transplantation, 17*, 1447–1454.

Matesanz, R., Miranda, B., & Felipe, C. (1994). Organ procurement in Spain: Impact of transplant coordination. *Clinical Transplantation, 8*, 281–286.

Medicina, C. F. D. (2017). *Resolução n°2173, de 23 de novembro de 2017* (240th ed.). Diário Oficial da União.

Medicina, C. F. D. (2019). In C. F. D. Medicina (Ed.), *Código de Ética Médica: Resolução CFM n°2217, de 27 de setembro de 2018, modificada pelas Resoluções CFM n°2.222/2018 e 2.226/2019*. Conselho Federal de Medicina.

ONT. (1999). *Meeting the organ shortage: An European consensus document. Newsletter Transplant*.

PNUD. (2020). *Relatório do Desenvolvimento Humano 2020*. Programa das Nações Unidas para o Desenvolvimento (PNUD).

República, P. D. (2017). *DECRETO N° 9.175, DE 18 DE OUTUBRO DE 2017*. Secretaria Geral, Subchefia para assuntos jurídicos.

Sheehy, E., Conrad, S. L., Brigham, L. E., Luskin, R., Weber, P., Eakin, M., Schkade, L., & Hunsicker, L. (2003). Estimating the number of potential organ donors in the United States. *The New England Journal of Medicine, 349*, 667–674.

Silveira, F. (2011). Transplantes no PR: há que melhorar. *Conselho Regional de Medicina do Paraná.*, 01/11/2011.

Tannous, L. A., Yazbek, V. M. C. Y., Giugni, J. R., Garbossa, M. C. P., & Camara, B. M. D. (2018). *Manual para notificação, diagnóstico de morte encefálica e manutenção do potencial doador de órgãos e tecidos*. Secretaria de Estado da Saúde do Paraná.

Vasconcelos, C. M., & Pasche, D. F. (2012). O SUS em perspectiva. In G. W. D. S. Campos (Ed.), *Tratado de Saúde Coletiva*. Hucitec.

Chapter 2
Pathway to Convert a Potential in an Actual Organ Donor

Donation Effectiveness

The identification of a potential donor triggers a series of processes to finalize the diagnostic protocol and confirm the brain death and hopefully the conversion. **Conversion** is the technical term used to describe a potential donor who becomes an actual donor.

The diagnostic confirmation, the analysis of potential medical counterindications, the family's authorization, donor's care, and organ-harvesting surgery are the elements that affect the donation's effectiveness.

The State Transplant Center developed a management flowchart (Tannous et al., 2018) that follows the brain death diagnosis (Fig. 2.1).

Within a limited time, sometimes a matter of a few hours, the family may receive confirmation of the brain death diagnosis and will eventually be approached with regard to organ donation.

Confirmation of Brain Death Diagnosis

The conduction of two clinical exams, the apnea test and an additional confirmation exam, is the necessary stages for diagnostic confirmation, a sequence of steps set by the legislation and documented by the State Transplant Center (Tannous et al., 2018).

Striving for the process transparency, the participation of physicians who are members of transplant teams is forbidden. Furthermore, two different physicians must conduct the clinical exams.

© The Author(s), under exclusive license to Springer Nature Switzerland AG 2022
F. Silveira, A. T. C. G. Badoch, *Effective Public Health Policy in Organ Donation*,
SpringerBriefs in Public Health, https://doi.org/10.1007/978-3-030-99288-0_2

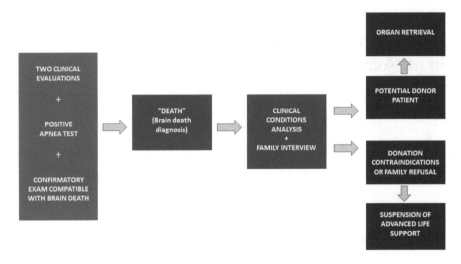

Fig. 2.1 Flowchart of conducts followed by brain death diagnosis

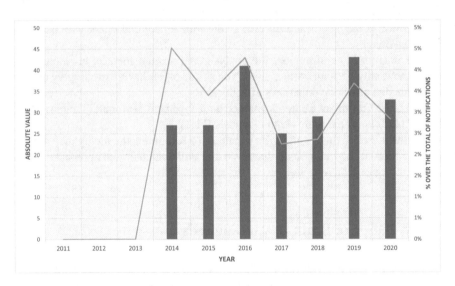

Fig. 2.2 Non-confirmation of brain death diagnosis – total and proportional numbers of all notifications

Given the vast set of clinical signs, which raise suspicion of the brain death diagnostic, it is unusual to diagnose non-confirmation by complementary examinations (Fig. 2.2). On average, non-confirmed diagnosis accounted for 3% of the reasons for not proceeding with a donation. It is an insufficiently representative cause in the set of reasons for non-conversion.

Medical Contraindications

There are few absolute contraindications for organ donation in the medical literature (EDQM, 2010) and legislation (BRASIL, 2017). They are related to some diseases of potential transmission to the donor, neoplasms, and uncontained infections. Often, they are not easily characterized, which highlights the relevance of being conducted by experienced physicians in the field, and never assigned to nonmedical technical or even higher-level professionals.

Despite few medical grounds, on average, they accounted for 20% of the causes for donation nonperformance (Fig. 2.3). Potential donors' age range increases (Badoch et al., 2021), and the policy culture of effective brain death diagnosis justifies these numbers.

In 2019 and 2020, the most common causes of donation disposal due to medical contraindication were uncontrolled active infectious diseases (sepsis), neoplasms, and coronavirus-positive serologies (Fig. 2.4).

It must be stressed that, at this stage of the process, which is the actual donation, the absolute donation contraindications are solely mentioned. The transplanting team must analyze the donor's/recipient's evaluation's relative contraindications after the donation has been made.

Family Authorization

The family's support is one of the greatest challenges of health professionals, which for brain death situations is developed by the CIHDOTT staff in cooperation with intensive care teams. This family-hospital interaction is considered one of the most

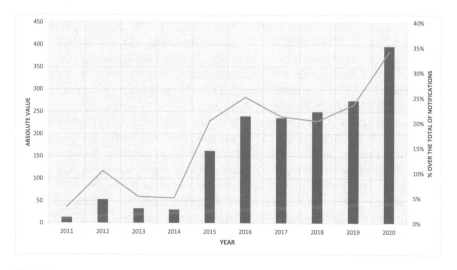

Fig. 2.3 Medical contraindications of the total and the proportional number of all notifications

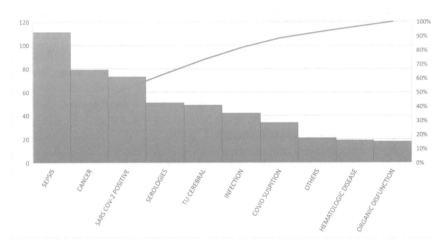

Fig. 2.4 Main reasons for medical contraindication in 2019–2020

relevant aspects of care, which impacts both during and after hospitalization (Gries et al., 2010). It was one of the major challenges faced throughout the reshaping of Paraná's system (Heberle, 2017).

The shared role of CIHDOTT/OPO in this context is vital, as the healthcare team itself finds this approach both challenging and distressing, often seen as an extra burden to the grieving family (Kentish-Barnes et al., 2019).

Nationwide, a donation requires the family's authorization (República, 1997). Identifying the anchor family member, the responsible one for making decisions, is one of the first steps in the process, which is not always easy. The anchor family member is not always related to direct family or marital status but might be religiously, socially, and culturally influenced. Only family members up to the second degree, including the spouse (República, 2017), can provide legal authorization.

Some aspects are the major influencers in the family's decision, such as the family member's previous opinion on organ donations (Traino et al., 2017). Unfortunately, this knowledge is not the rule. The accurate and complete information provision, a suitable place for communication, adequate language techniques, perception of assurance of respect, and care to the body are all complementary to the family decision (Kentish-Barnes et al., 2019).

A fundamental part of embracement is proper communication, yet embracement is more than this. Language techniques can be learned and taught, but communication involves more than this: perception of sincerity, cooperation, honesty, and listening are fundamental. We live in a social reality where social support such as resting place, transportation, clothing, and food is often of greater importance.

On average, the family's lack of authorization outcomes in 21% of a non-donation. This number is progressively decreasing and is currently at 14% (Fig. 2.5).

Regarding the reasons for not performing a donation, family refusal represents from 5.7% to 41.4% in European (Transplant, 2014) countries, from 23% to 66.6%

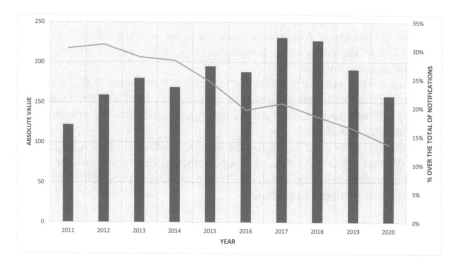

Fig. 2.5 Absolute and relative progression of family's refusals

in South America (Transplant, 2014), 45% in the United States (Siminoff et al., 2001), and 42% in Brazil (ABTO, 2020). **With system's improvement, Paraná managed to reduce this average found in the west.**

It is possible to see that the donation's authorization involves multiple facts that ultimately reflect a humane treatment since the beginning of the pathological condition. It entails an accessible healthcare system, an early approach, and explanation of what is happening to the family member, as well as a feeling of security in the treatment provided. A decrease in family negative rates is indicative of the quality of care provided by the involved agents and the unified health system.

Donor's Care

Brain death brings significant consequences for the balance and for the homeostasis of our organism. The disruption of control processes, hormone release, and hemodynamic maintenance happen to a greater or lower degree in these patients. In addition to this, there are the patient's characteristics, as prior illnesses or those that resulted from the brain death etiology itself (Tannous, 2019).

Donor's care is the set of medical and pharmacological interventions that aim to restore or delay the pathophysiological consequences of brain death and must be initiated as soon as the suspected diagnosis is made (Tannous et al., 2018), which is a crucial stage for organ donations.

Improper care may result in cardiac arrest events, which definitively makes the use of the organs unfeasible. Initially, an important cause for non-donations in the state (Gois et al., 2017), the presence – from 2014 onward – of the intensive care physician role at the State Transplant Center, in constant contact with the notifying hospitals, has resulted in a significant reduction of the problem. Previously responsible for 15% of the non-donation causes, currently, cardiac arrest is responsible for 5% of the reasons (Fig. 2.6).

It is not always possible to achieve or maintain hemodynamic stability. In these situations, if the family has consented to the donation, local collection teams are promptly actioned to separately collect kidneys, to maximize the availability of organs for transplantation.

Proper care, apart from enhancing the number of effective donors, impacts the use of donated organs. Patients with poor hemodynamic conditions for several hours lead to organ suffering, which affects its possibility of use and even its proper functionality in posttransplant periods.

Donor's Conversion

To transform a potential donor into an actual donor is the conclusion of one of the transplant system's stages. As previously outlined, this moment shapes the interaction of several factors directly affected by the OPO-CIHDOTT's performance as this interaction makes things happen.

Assembling all the reasons that influence the transformation of a potential donor into an actual donor, over the decade, we realize the global impact of the system's reorganization (Fig. 2.7).

The reduction in the family refusal area and cardiac arrest was followed by the virtual disappearance of other reasons that led to the non-conversion of a donation.

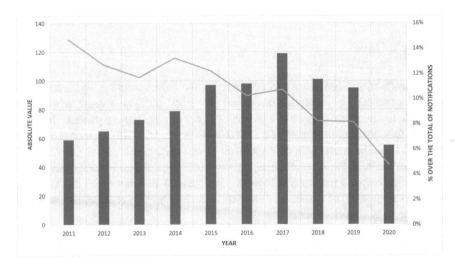

Fig. 2.6 Absolute and proportional growth of potential donor's cardiac arrest

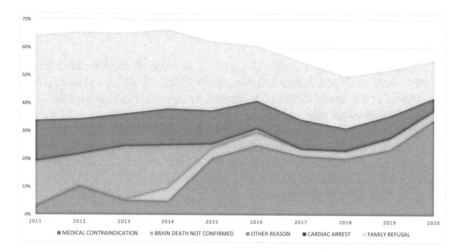

Fig. 2.7 An overview of the decade's reasons for donations' failure of potential organ donors

Table 2.1 Percentual value of non-conversion reasons in relation to the absolute number of notifications

	2011	2012	2013	2014	2015	2016	2017	2018	2019	2020	Total
Medical contraindication	3%	10%	5%	5%	20%	25%	21%	20%	24%	34%	20%
Non-confirmation of brain death diagnosis	0%	0%	0%	5%	3%	4%	2%	2%	4%	3%	3%
Other reasons	16%	11%	19%	15%	2%	1%	0%	0%	0%	0%	4%
Cardiac arrest	15%	13%	12%	13%	12%	10%	11%	8%	8%	5%	10%
Family's refusal	30%	31%	29%	28%	25%	20%	21%	18%	16%	14%	21%
Total	64%	66%	65%	66%	62%	61%	55%	50%	52%	56%	58%

The disappearance of other reasons resulted from the effort to detail and specify the causes, carry out interventions, and improve quality.

Medical contraindications were the only area that expanded. This expansion resulted from accepting the brain death diagnosis culture and the potential donors' age pyramid expansion (Table 2.1).

The decade analysis demonstrates a reduction in the frequency of the range of reasons, which result in a donor's non-conversion. Nevertheless, an average of 58% of notifications does not result in an actual donor, a rate that initially reached 66% and reached its best – 50% – in 2018.

The conversion frequency has a considerably wide range reported in the literature, from 15 to 67% (Garcia, 2000; Sheehy et al., 2003), and the average in the state of Paraná – of 42% – within this range.

Besides providing humanized and proper care for the 58% who do not become actual donors, this measure results in a spending reduction of ICU daily fees and therapeutic resources of the Brazilian National Health System (SUS).

In situations where brain death diagnosis is confirmed and donation is not per-formed, life support is withdrawn, with no ethical (Medicina, 2007) or legal (República, 2017) implications.

Identifying and giving a correct diagnosis to brain death patients, even though not all of them result in a donation, foster a positive and life-saving cycle, which we can observe in the rising number of performed transplants (Fig. 2.8 and Table 2.2).

The effective donor ultimately plays the role of a quality parameter for the entire health system, as it involves access, treatment, diagnosis, and adequate care.

Once concluded, the stage for the conversion of a potential donor is followed by the organization of the organ-collecting surgery, histocompatibility tests, recipient ranking, and distribution logistics stages. The State Transplant Center's 24-hour on-call sector coordinates these stages.

System Logistics Center

The State Transplant Center's operation sector is based in Curitiba, works 24 hours a day, and operates as a system's "hub." It bridges the gap between the notifying OPOs and the CIHDOTTs, histocompatibility laboratories, tissue banks, and trans-plant teams.

Donor's data is received and checked, and the potential receptor's rank is created according to the computerized system of the National Transplant System. Each agency has its distribution particularities, although always following technical and transparent criteria (BRASIL, 2009).

After the classification, the transplant team's contact phase with the patients begins. The logistics organization of team's transport and organ distribution

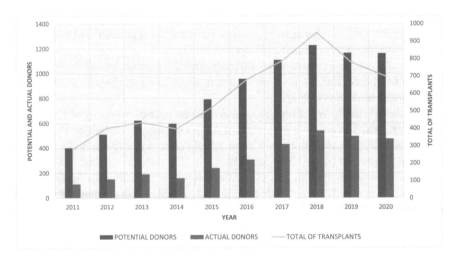

Fig. 2.8 Rise in the number of transplants regarding the culture of brain death notification

Table 2.2 Number of potential donors, effective donors, and transplants

	Potential donors	Effective donors	Effective donation pmp	Total of transplants
2011	401	111	10.7	279
2012	511	151	14.5	401
2013	623	191	18.3	433
2014	597	159	16.6	397
2015	793	241	21.7	517
2016	956	307	30.9	678
2017	1110	432	38	786
2018	1228	540	47.7	949
2019	1166	497	43.8	778
2020	1162	475	41.5	698

Pmp per million population

considers the geography, weather conditions, sort of dislocation, attendance of single or multiple teams, and surgery's surgery starting time.

The transport of the obtained and stored organs and teams that retrieve them is performed by land or air. The land route uses state vehicles and drivers. Air transport is conducted with the support of the Military House of the State Government, using planes or helicopters. For transports between states, there is the Brazilian Air Force support, enabled after the federal government's decree (Brasil, 2016). Commercial air transport has a unique way of supporting the system transporting teams or organs through their scheduled routes, according to seat availability and free of charge (ABEAR, 2014).

The distance from the transplant center where the transplant will be performed affects the chosen transport method – regarding the heart, lung, and liver – weather conditions, the donor's hemodynamic stability and the availability of air travel, and deadline that the family wishes and the deadline that the family wishes for the delivery of the donor's body. Despite being a supportive and available system, aircraft are not for the exclusive use of the State Transplant System.

As observed, the logistic is multifactorial; however, it seeks to meet two requirements, hemodynamic stability and the family's wish to follow the agreed delivery time of the donor's body.

Once the ranking and logistical definition are concluded; the organ extraction surgery is scheduled. The organs that will be transplanted are determined after the organ extraction surgery according to their anatomic and physiologic conditions. Upon the surgery conclusion, with proper reconstitution of the body, the transplant center/OPO/CIHDOTT helps the family with funeral arrangements.

For transplants that require histocompatibility, it's necessary to conduct tests – the kidney and pancreas; tissue samples (spleen and lymph nodes) are sent to specialized laboratories, which will later determine the receivers' classification.

In heart, lung, and liver transplants, these organs are immediately sent to the destination hospitals as soon as the organ extraction surgery finishes. After the removed organs are cooled and stored, there are a limited time window – hours – for the proper transplantation in the receivers.

Thus, the activity of the system's logistics center must strive for proactivity and agility, ensuring the safety and traceability of all actions involved in the notification, donation, extraction, and distribution of organs for transplantation.

References

ABEAR. (2014). *Asas do Bem* [Online]. Associação Brasileira das Empresas Aéreas. Available: https://www.abear.com.br/sobre/responsabilidade-social/. Accessed 15 June 2021.

ABTO. (2020). In V. D. Garcia (Ed.), *RBT - Registro Brasileiro de Transplantes*. ABTO - Associação Brasileira de Transplante de Órgãos.

Badoch, A. T., Silveira, F., Von Stein, A., & Giugni, J. (2021). Mudança no padrão demográfico dos doadores de órgãos no Estado do Paraná de 2011 a 2019. *Revista de Saúde Pública do Paraná, 4*.

BRASIL. (2009). In M. D. Saúde (Ed.), *Portaria n°2600, de 21 de outubro de 2009*. Diário Oficial da União.

BRASIL. (2016). Decreto 8783/16 | Decreto n° 8.783, de 6 de junho de 2016.

BRASIL. (2017). *Portaria de Consolidação n°4, de 28 de setembro de 2017*. Ministério da Saúde.

EDQM. (2010). *Guide to the safety and quality assurance for the transplantation of organs, tissues and cells*. Strasbourg, France.

Garcia, V. D. (2000). *Por uma política de transplantes no Brasil*. São Paulo.

Gois, R., Galdino, M., Pissinati, P., Pimentel, R., Carvalho, M., & Haddad, M. (2017). Efetividade do processo de doação de órgãos para transplantes. *Acta Paulista de Enfermagem [online], 30*, 621–627.

Gries, C. J., Engelberg, R. A., Kross, E. K., Zatzick, D., Nielsen, E. L., Downey, L., & Curtis, J. R. (2010). Predictors of symptoms of posttraumatic stress and depression in family members after patient death in the ICU. *Chest, 137*, 280–287.

Heberle, L. C. (2017). *Atuação do enfermeiro no processo de doação de órgãos: entrevista familiar*. Universidade Federal do Paraná.

Kentish-Barnes, N., Siminoff, L. A., Walker, W., Urbanski, M., Charpentier, J., Thuong, M., Sarti, A., Shemie, S. D., & Azoulay, E. (2019). A narrative review of family members' experience of organ donation request after brain death in the critical care setting. *Intensive Care Medicine, 45*, 331–342.

Medicina, C. F. D. (2007). *RESOLUÇÃO CFM N° 1.826/2007*. Diário Oficial da União.

República, P. D. (1997). *LEI N° 9.434, DE 4 DE FEVEREIRO DE 1997*. In: Jurídicos, C. C., S. P. a. (Eds.).

República, P. D. (2017). *DECRETO N° 9.175, DE 18 DE OUTUBRO DE 2017*. Secretaria Geral, Subchefia para assuntos jurídicos.

Sheehy, E., Conrad, S. L., Brigham, L. E., Luskin, R., Weber, P., Eakin, M., Schkade, L., & Hunsicker, L. (2003). Estimating the number of potential organ donors in the United States. *The New England Journal of Medicine, 349*, 667–674.

Siminoff, L. A., Gordon, N., Hewlett, J., & Arnold, R. M. (2001). Factors influencing families' consent for donation of solid organs for transplantation. *JAMA, 286*, 71–77.

Tannous, L. A. (2019). *Benefício clínico, laboratorial e histológico de uma estratégia otimizada de manutenção do potencial doador de órgãos - modelo experimental em coelhos*. Pontifícia Universidade Católica do Paraná.

Tannous, L. A., Yazbek, V. M. C. Y., Giugni, J. R., Garbossa, M. C. P., & Camara, B. M. D. (2018). *Manual para notificação, diagnóstico de morte encefálica e manutenção do potencial doador de órgãos e tecidos*. Secretaria de Estado da Saúde do Paraná.

Traino, H. M., Molisani, A. J., & Siminoff, L. A. (2017). Regional differences in communication process and outcomes of requests for solid organ donation. *American Journal of Transplantation, 17*, 1620–1627.

Transplant, C. O. E. S. N. (2014). In R. Matesanz (Ed.), *International figures on donation an transplantation - 2013*. Council of Europe's Newsletter Transplant.

Chapter 3
Strengthening the Donation Process

Growth Enhancers

The structuring of the diagnosis and donor converting network must be strengthened on several fronts, whether by maximizing the use of donated organs, continued education procedures aiming to improve family support, detailed attention to the process financial viability, setting up a network of histocompatibility laboratories essential to perform transplants, and developing awareness campaigns. Each of the stages was a foundation for the overall system's expansion.

Expanding the Borders

The goal to achieve a full diagnosis of brain death had to be followed by a shift in paradigms regarding the possibility to use organs from identified potential donors. At the very beginning of the system's redesign, high rejection rates of potential donors were found due to reasons that lacked further scientific evidence. This discard often happened on a local scale, whether on the notifying hospital or OPO or else at the State Transplant Center before it reached the scrutiny of the transplant team and was conducted by not specialists in the field. The system had to understand and mature the use of expanded criteria donors.

Unlike the so-called standard donors – young, healthy, brain-dead trauma patients – the expanded criteria donors fall into an older age group and/or with comorbidities. The evolution of transplant medicine itself was responsible for expanding the horizons of the use of organs.

Among the diverse transplant procedures, whether of the heart, liver, pancreas, lungs, or kidneys, the advances of surgical techniques, intensive care, rejection control, and proper screening of receivers led the procedure's risk per se to prove to be

F. Silveira, A. T. C. G. Badoch, *Effective Public Health Policy in Organ Donation*, SpringerBriefs in Public Health, https://doi.org/10.1007/978-3-030-99288-0_3

lower than the risk of keeping the patient on a waiting list, which explains the maximized use of such a precious resource – the donated organ.

It must be stressed that to receive an organ from an expanded criteria donor does not imply receiving a damaged organ. The decision-making chain for the use of an expanded criteria donor organ involves an evaluation of the recipient-donor relation. That is, the donor characteristics need to be "matched" with the recipient characteristics. In a given donation offer, an expanded organ donor may not be suitable for a specific receiver, yet in the following donation, this receiver may be perfectly matched. The final decision of whether or not to use an organ is essentially technical, which is always up to the transplant team.

Two steps were initially designed: first, to refute the idea of limiting the donation based on the donor's age and to transfer the use of organ decision to transplant teams, in the event of relative contraindications. The second step was to have the presence of intensive care specialized physicians in the transplant center, who are capable to distinguish the presence of total donation contraindications.

Throughout the decade, there has been an expansion of donors' base in the state, with a significant average age increase (Badoch et al., 2021). There has been a 33.7% increase in donors' numbers within the 50–64 age group and a 91.58% increase in the 65–79 age group. Within the youngest donors' group, 18–34 years old, a 40.4% reduction was identified (Fig. 3.1). It is worth pointing out that the ageing of the population basis is an outcome of higher diagnostic effectiveness, as well as due to the society's human development, which results in an aged population with a decrease in youth mortality due to external causes (violence, accidents of traffic).

The shift of the age pattern was followed by a change of the etiology of brain deaths (Fig. 3.2). Previously mainly traumatic, stroke became the most frequent

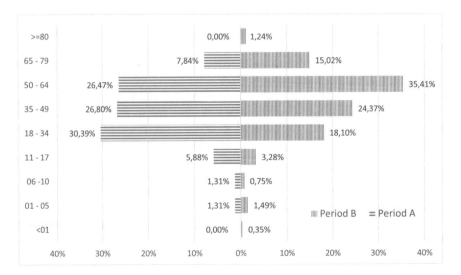

Fig. 3.1 Alteration of the effective donors' age pattern of Paraná. (Period A (2011–2014) and Period B (2015–2019))

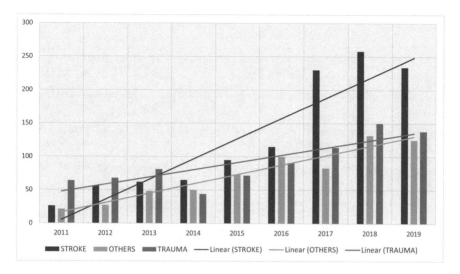

Fig. 3.2 Alteration of brain death etiology occurrence

etiology (46.35%), a pattern shift equally observed in other populations (Meers et al., 2009).

With ageing and strokes prevailing, it is natural to observe a decline in the number of organs used by each effective donor. While regarding young, healthy donors, it is common to use, from a single donor, the heart, lungs, kidneys, pancreas, and liver, while regarding older donors, the organ ratio usage decreases.

This alteration in donor's characteristics, through the use of expanded criteria, has been reported in the liver (Routh et al., 2013) and kidney (Aubert et al., 2015) transplants, with limited use due to the need for technological resources, which are still unavailable in our country, when it comes to heart and lung transplants.

The expanded criteria donors' use is only appropriate for specific receiver subgroups, likely to impact outcomes (Goldberg et al., 2015).

This expected pattern, the ratio drop of transplant/actual donor, owed to the demographic base expansion of the donor, contrasts with the rising trend of the transplant line per million population (Fig. 3.3 and Table 3.1).

The opposite trend of the lines strengthens the system's overall ultimate goal, to save the highest number of lives. **Undoubtedly, the donor's base expansion policy can benefit an ever-growing number of patients**.

Continuing Education Programs

Training people involved in the identification process and donation execution stages is one of the most significant achievements of the Paraná State Transplant System. These pieces of training were gradually developed, formulated, and reformulated

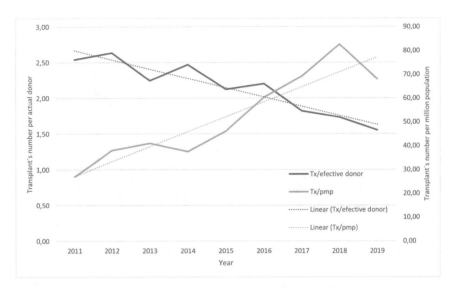

Fig. 3.3 Relation of transplants per actual donor and per million population

Table 3.1 Relation of transplants per actual donor and per million population

	2011	2012	2013	2014	2015	2016	2017	2018	2019
Total of transplants	282	398	429	393	512	674	778	935	771
Effective donations	111	151	191	159	241	306	427	540	497
Transplant/effective donor ratio	2.54	2.64	2.25	2.47	2.12	2.20	1.82	1.73	1.55
Population (×1000) of Paraná	10,439	10,439	10,444	10,444	11,081	11,163	11,242	11,320	11,348
Transplant/pmp ratio	27.01	38.13	41.08	37.63	46.21	60.38	69.20	82.60	67.94

according to the emerged needs of the several different realities of the state's OPOs and CIHDOTTs.

These courses and training rely on State Transplant Center's (CET) medical and nursing planning and involve brain death diagnosis, donor's care, support and communication techniques, surgical room coordination, and revenue of the hospital's donation procedures.

This actual continuing education program takes place at state, regional. and local levels. State meetings, known as CIHDOTT's State Meetings – ENCIHDOTTs – acted as long-range cannons for the propagation of information, courses as well as training, in addition to the integration and interaction of the system's direct responsible parties. The manifestation of pride and joy for joining a collaborative work was visible during these meetings.

The interaction of the CET team with the ICU health team, at first in *loco*, supported the diagnosis of brain death instructing, prejudice dissipation, and CIHDOTTs' work confidence building.

Striving to prove their expertise in the ongoing work, the state ICUs' responsible physicians have come to consider the CET's intensive care unit and the CIHDOTTs' nurses as sources for assistance in the brain death identification task, rather than additional sources of trouble. **This interaction was a cornerstone in the development and consolidation of the brain death diagnosis culture**. This work not only takes place in technical or practical formal courses but also at the bedside, assisting in the process.

Similarly, welcoming and communication courses were held in more restricted clusters, engaging fewer CIHDOTTs, larger meetings, and *on-site* monitoring of hundreds of family approaches.

As the reception and communication process takes place throughout several stages within the brain death diagnosis process, State Transplant System keeps a direct and active communication channel among its members. This channel has proven to be of unparalleled value, given that people's interactions, experience sharing, approach methods, and dispute settlement are discussed within the family's approach, therefore increasing the system's effectiveness.

Given that the system is decentralized, the OPO coordinators can more effectively detect local problems and request the CET's educational intervention.

The intensive care medical team can increase the quality of the potential donor's care, under the charge of the several ICUs in the state, through telephone contact and by incentivizing to follow the checklists. Educational videos, brain death diagnosis local courses, and potential donors' care have been taught over the years.

The educational methodology of local courses, *on-site* intervention, and telephone support became physically exhausting as the demand increased. Due to the significant territory extension, Curitiba team's availability in all health regional offices and CIHDOTTs in the state was becoming increasingly more difficult. The system has adjusted with the introduction of local instructors, who then began to deliver courses in their respective geographical areas, an additional element that has contributed to maintaining the continuing education principle. The continuing education principle is essential due to the natural turnover of the CIHDOTT team members.

Formal courses are sponsored by Paraná's public health school through the payment of instructors' hourly fees, combined with partnerships with institutions that deliver the courses, which provide the remaining needs accordingly to each case.

Funding

In 2011, Paraná State's Government, via the state's health secretary, implemented a funding program (HOSPSUS) for public and charity hospitals that provide services to the unified health system. Aiming for quality and conclusive service, it implemented metrics that, according to their fulfilment, linked funds' transfer from the program (Paraná, 2011). The State Transplant System has raised awareness among the state government concerning the importance of the brain death diagnosis as a quality indicator for the system, resulting in the presence of an active CIHDOTT as one of the elements linked to the funds' transfer. The State Transplant System brought to the state government's attention the importance of the brain death diagnosis as a quality indicator for the system, resulting in the incorporation of an active CIHDOTT presence as one of the elements linked to the funds' transfer.

To eliminate the subjective nature of an active CIHDOTT definition, the State Transplant System developed (Duarte, 2019) and implemented an Evaluation Manual of the Performance of Intra-Hospital Organ and Tissue Donation for Transplants (SET/PR, 2018), which established objective criteria for this qualification. CIHDOTT's incorporation into HOSPSUS – which has quarterly evaluations – was a system's major achievement and contributed to financing State Transplant System.

The brain death detection process involves operational and human resource costs. At the initial redesigning of the system, hospitals lack of charging for provided services was a hampering fact of the system's implementation. Due to a lack of knowledge, hospitals did not profit from the stages of the process funded by SUS. Besides pursuing providers to implement the CIHDOTTS, the State Transplant Center has prepared a manual (SET/PR, 2017) and assigned a human resources section to guide all notifying hospitals' billing stages.

Genetics and Histocompatibility Laboratory Network

Humans have a gene complex – called HLA – that encodes proteins associated with tissue rejection. Knowing the chain of these genes enables us to understand the mechanisms involved in graft rejection and maintenance, enabling therapeutic improvements, such as better selection of the receiver/donor binomial or immunosuppressive medications.

Hence, knowledge of this gene chain – the HLA classification – is crucial in organ or tissue transplants. Regarding solid organs from deceased donors' circumstances, the classification is performed using a blood sample from the receiver, which remains in the labs and, on the occasion of the donation, is compared with the donor's HLA classification, contributing to a more accurate compatibility definition. This process happens 24 hours a day.

In living donor transplants, the analysis is electively performed prior to the transplant; this practice is most commonly found in marrow and kidney transplants.

This lab network, which has undergone readjustments over the decade (BRASIL, 2012), is also responsible for the Voluntary Bone Marrow Donors Registry (REDOME) maintenance used in transplants of hematopoietic stem cells with non-related donors for therapeutic purposes.

Currently, the state has a well-structured and satisfactory network to meet the demand, composed of labs qualified to perform serological or molecular histocompatibility tests, as well as to register voluntary marrow donors, spread out in Curitiba's counties, Londrina and Maringá.

Awareness Campaigns

Emotions rule organ donations, not logical and analytical reasoning. When the family denies the donation, this reflects either a desire expressed by the deceased or unawareness of their desire, in most cases (Silveira, 2012).

The policy of the State Transplant System sought to open flow and encourage awareness campaigns regarding this matter, however, without the use of public resources in advertising campaigns.

The creation of the logo in 2014 – *Organ donation. Talk about it* (see Fig. 3.4) – seeks to draw attention to the importance of discussing the topic within the family, which is recognized as relevant decision-making-supporting element for grieving families. The logo has received the title of state campaign, not the government's, and its promotion has been conducted and supported by tens of partners across the private sector (Paraná, 2021).

The media coverage to suppress the organ donation myths related to donor's age limitations, associated diseases, additional funeral costs following the donation, body mutilation, anonymity, the fairness of organ donation and distribution systems, and the assurance of a correct diagnosis has frequent topics of awareness messages or campaigns (Silveira, 2020).

Fig. 3.4 Awareness campaign logo

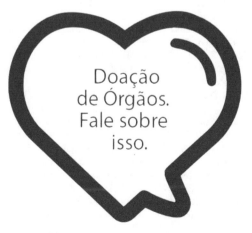

"Organ donation. Talk about it."

These campaigns always intensify in September, especially in the last week, as the 27th is National Organ and Tissue Donors' Day, and the month is called "Green September."

This line of approach – not spending public funds on awareness campaigns – was based on evidence that they have a temporary impact on donation rates (Frates et al., 2006), and therefore, they should be conducted in partnership with the private system. The distribution of public resources, which are always limited, must be addressed to active search, diagnosis, and family welcoming activities.

References

Aubert, O., Kamar, N., Vernerey, D., Viglietti, D., Martinez, F., Duong-Van-Huyen, J. P., Eladari, D., Empana, J. P., Rabant, M., Verine, J., Rostaing, L., Congy, N., Guilbeau-Frugier, C., Mourad, G., Garrigue, V., Morelon, E., Giral, M., Kessler, M., Ladriere, M., … Loupy, A. (2015). Long term outcomes of transplantation using kidneys from expanded criteria donors: Prospective, population based cohort study. *BMJ, 351*, h3557.

Badoch, A. T., Silveira, F., Von Stein, A., & Giugni, J. (2021). Mudança no padrão demográfico dos doadores de órgãos no Estado do Paraná de 2011 a 2019. *Revista de Saúde Pública do Paraná, 4*.

BRASIL. (2012). In M. D. Saúde (Ed.), *Portaria n°844, de 2 de maio de 2012*. Ministério da Saúde - Gabinete do Ministro.

Duarte, G. F. (2019). *Construção de processo avaliativo para comissões intra-hospitalares de transplante*. Universidade Estadual de Maringá.

Frates, J., Bohrer, G. G., & Thomas, D. (2006). Promoting organ donation to Hispanics: The role of the media and medicine. *Journal of Health Communication, 11*, 683–698.

Goldberg, D. S., French, B., Abt, P. L., & Gilroy, R. K. (2015). Increasing the number of organ transplants in the United States by optimizing donor authorization rates. *American Journal of Transplantation, 15*, 2117–2125.

Meers, C., Van Raemdonck, D., Van Gelder, F., Van Hees, D., Desschans, B., De Roey, J., Vanhaecke, J., Pirenne, J., & Transplantation, U. Z. L. C. F. (2009). Change in donor profile influenced the percentage of organs transplanted from multiple organ donors. *Transplantation Proceedings, 41*, 572–575.

Paraná, G. D. E. D. (2011). In S. D. Saúde (Ed.), *Resolução SESA n° 0172/2011*. Diário Oficial do Estado n° 8510 de 19/07/11.

Paraná, S. E. D. T. D. (2021). *Empresas, Instituições e Entidades Parceiras*. [Online]. Available: http://www.paranatransplantes.pr.gov.br/Pagina/Empresas-Instituicoes-e-Entidades-Parceiras. Accessed 14 June 2021.

Routh, D., Naidu, S., Sharma, S., Ranjan, P., & Godara, R. (2013). Changing pattern of donor selection criteria in deceased donor liver transplant: A review of literature. *Journal of Clinical and Experimental Hepatology, 3*, 337–346.

SET/PR. (2017). *Manual de cobrança de procedimentos de ações relacionadas à doação de órgãos e transplantes para hospitais SUS e não SUS*. Sistema Estadual de Transplantes do Paraná.

SET/PR. (2018). *Manual de Avaliação da Atuação da Comissão Intra-Hospitalar de Doação de Órgãos e Tecidos para Transplante - CIHDOTT*. Sistema Estadual de Transplantes do Paraná.

Silveira, F. (2012). *Conscientizar para salvar*. Gazeta do Povo.

Silveira, F. (2020). *Setembro Verde - Vamos falar sobre a doação de órgãos para transplante*. Tribuna do Paraná.

Chapter 4
Access, Outcome, and Monitoring of Transplants

Transplants

Organ transplantation has a passionate history of extraordinary success in modern medicine. In the ten years, 205,233 Brazilians had the opportunity to improve quality and/or extend their life span through organ transplants (the heart, lung, kidney, pancreas, liver) or tissue (cornea) obtained via deceased donors (ABTO, 2020).

This medicine area faces a series of challenges and obstacles, related to genetic characteristics identification (histocompatibility), the required use of immunosuppressants, infectious disease exposure, and evolution of surgical, anesthesia, and intensive care techniques. These are technical issues that, thanks to the efforts of outstanding scientists and physicians, have been tackled and led to modern advances capable of benefiting thousands of patients, even in countries with socioeconomic inequalities so obvious as in our own.

The previously listed characteristics alone already rank transplants in a unique position, but their interface is much broader. Its increasing therapeutic effectiveness combined with the ageing society organ failure increase uncovers the organ failure issue prominently. This issue raises a series of medical, bioethical, and health discussions among authorities regarding brain death, donation permission, inter vivos donation, xenotransplantation, and organ allocation – only mentioning just a few of them – often involving emotional issues that deeply move public opinion.

Transplants have several recommendations, and the mythical image of an end-stage procedure performed on the deathbed is not true. Some have more significant impacts on life quality (corneas, bones, tendons), others on life expectancy (kidneys, pancreas), while others impact life span significantly (the heart, lung, liver). The 5-year liver and heart transplant survival rate in Paraná State has reached 60% in five years. Regarding untreated diseases, these don't permit the survival of the majority of patients for more than a few months. Comparatively, the 5-year overall

© The Author(s), under exclusive license to Springer Nature Switzerland AG 2022
F. Silveira, A. T. C. G. Badoch, *Effective Public Health Policy in Organ Donation*,
SpringerBriefs in Public Health, https://doi.org/10.1007/978-3-030-99288-0_4

survival for breast, intestine, and prostate cancers is 52%, 46%, and 51%, respectively (Instituto Nacional do Câncer, 2021).

Aiming to increase the organ supply, Paraná State Transplant System also strived to organize and streamline other stages and players in this complex process.

Treatment Access

Understanding that democratic access, as recommended by the single health system, is supposed to be available to all Paraná citizens, the design of the State Transplant System prioritized the increase of outpatient and emergency access to transplant centers.

Availability of metrics access to treatment within the scope of SUS, aiming at no differentiation with private assistance network, was implemented along with transplant centers through the adoption of referral flows and attentiveness to the access of the system for patients from outside of Paraná (Paraná, 2018).

Hospitals and Transplant Teams

The results shown following the first years of the system's redesign contributed to motivating the teams, which assisted in implementing the project to increase the number of donations. The targeted donor's base expansion and use of expanded criteria donors echoed in the teams, which led to a progressive increase in the transplants' number performed in the state.

The organization of treatment access, organ collection availability, the establishment of routine protocols and constitution, and the operation of technical chambers were sequential steps of the system's reorganization.

A total of 147 teams in different hospitals and laboratories responsible for organ and tissue transplants are currently licensed throughout the State of Paraná. New accreditations were granted and others revoked, according to epidemiology criteria of need and commitment to the system (Fig. 4.1).

Waiting List

The single technical registry, known as the waiting list, is the Ministry of Health's computerized system that keeps a record of all patients in need of a transplant. It is supplied by transplant teams, responsible for inserting patients' data under their therapeutic responsibility, and managed by the State Transplant System. The system is transparent and follows specific ranking rules to each agency determined by

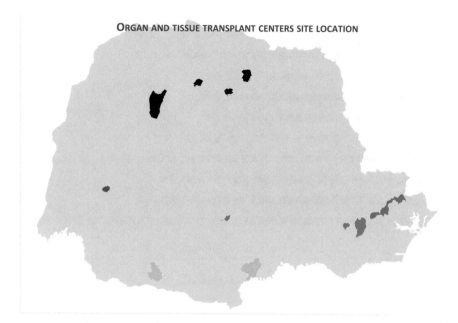

ORGAN AND TISSUE TRANSPLANT CENTERS SITE LOCATION

Fig. 4.1 Organ and tissue transplant centers' site location

legislation, and the patient has access to electronic consulting of their data (BRASIL, 2017).

Although it is nationwide, the patient is registered in the hospital's waiting list of the state where the treatment is provided. The patient can't be listed in more than one list in different states at the same time.

The graphic evolution of the waiting list during the last decade of the State Transplant System reveals a concavity pattern, annually including roughly 1500–200 patients (Fig. 4.2).

Although the design is mostly affected by larger numeric lists – the kidney and liver – it behaves similarly for all organs. As the system is gradually structured and the availability of organs and transplants increases, we have noticed a decrease – not elimination – in the number of patients on the waiting list, followed by a further increase associated with a subsequent increase (Table 4.1).

Despite having a dynamic character – patients enter and leave continuously – the graphic depiction has analytical value.

The waiting list length is affected by three factors: the patient's access to treatment, the availability of organs for transplantation, and transplant medicine. Although it seems unquestionable that increasing the number of donors can solve the problem of organ shortage, the reality is not so simple.

It is prudent to point out that the waiting list of organs that do not have an efficient replacement by artificial or pharmacological means has its growth limited by the mortality of these diseases, which results in undesirable waiting list mortality.

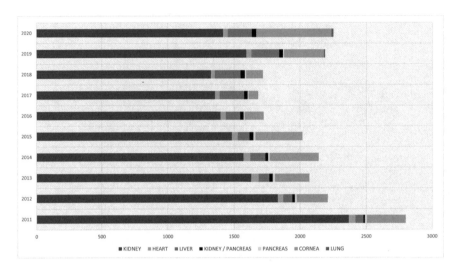

Fig. 4.2 Annual tendency of the transplant waiting list

Table 4.1 Number of patients in the waiting list for deceased organ or tissue donation

	2011	2012	2013	2014	2015	2016	2017	2018	2019	2020
Kidney	2367	1832	1630	1571	1482	1396	1354	1323	1593	1416
Heart	49	41	55	51	45	39	34	29	38	35
Liver	61	69	83	115	89	111	188	197	211	184
Kidney/pancreas	12	19	26	21	30	26	27	33	30	34
Pancreas	15	15	17	13	15	8	7	9	8	2
Cornea	293	233	259	369	357	144	72	127	301	566
Lung	0	0	0	0	0	0	0	0	8	15
Total	2797	2209	2070	2140	2018	1724	1682	1718	2189	2252

An effective and active transplant system – such as in Paraná – sought to ensure that the patient has access to treatment, eased by a universal public health system in place, and it intervened in the availability of organs for transplantation, therefore in the first two variables that comprise the waiting list.

The transplant system cannot control the third variable that impacts the waiting list, which is transplant medicine.

Thus, as transplant medicine grows and becomes more effective and safer, it inevitably requires more organs. More referrals are acknowledged, the urge for multiple transplants arises, and an inevitable condition is always present, the rejection of transplanted organs (Manzei, 2016).

Despite many significant improvements over the past decades, medicine cannot 100% effectively control the rejection process. This process, for some organs, ends up back feeding the system, increasing re-transplants and consequently the demand for more organs.

Thus, it is necessary to view the solid organ transplant waiting list as an issue to be managed, though not eliminated, since this is not possible in a brain-dead donor system.

A waiting list with constant patients' inflow and outflow, in a system, such as Paraná, with an appropriate quantity of donations, mirrors the system's health itself more than a disease.

The Beneficiated

To provide treatment to patients is the goal of the entire system. Dozens of diseases result in organ failure that eventually requires a transplant. Transplants aim to increase life prospects and quality, and each type of organ and tissue transplant has its characteristics.

Patients and family members when confronted with transplant diagnosis and indication express concern universally, but what about the donor? Without a donor, there is no transplant and no better chances. Brain-dead donors are essential living donors that are much more restricted and unfeasible to supply all needs.

Regarding solid organ transplants, 5644 transplants were performed in the state from 2011 to 2020, roughly 564 transplants per year or 1.54 transplants per day. Transplants with the highest number of performed procedures were liver and kidney transplants (Fig. 4.3 and Table 4.2).

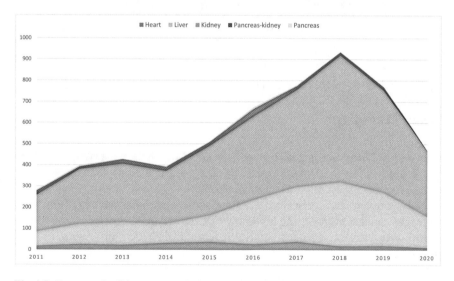

Fig. 4.3 Progress of solid organ transplants number performed

Table 4.2 Number of organ transplants performed

Year	Heart	Liver	Kidney	Pancreas-kidney	Pancreas	Total
2011	18	67	172	21	4	282
2012	26	95	259	12	6	398
2013	23	106	277	21	2	429
2014	32	91	249	19	2	393
2015	38	125	328	18	3	512
2016	27	209	394	36	8	674
2017	39	259	458	18	4	778
2018	19	302	598	15	1	935
2019	20	252	482	16	1	771
2020	11	147	308	4	2	472

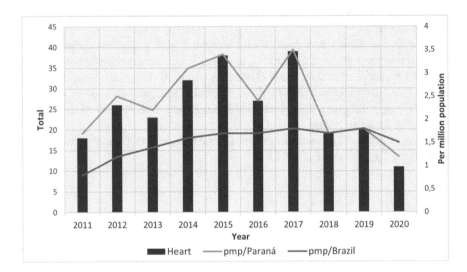

Fig. 4.4 Absolute and proportional heart transplant progress. (*pmp* per million population)

Heart Transplant

A total of 253 heart transplants were performed, of which the most common indication is heart failure – when the patient has fatigue, palpitations, breathlessness, or cardiogenic pain upon minimal physical effort.

The procedure has maintained absolute and proportional numbers (Fig. 4.4), above the national average, and is currently performed in six centers.

In 1-year, heart transplant's survival reaches 75.46% and, in 5 years, 66.86% (Fig. 4.5).

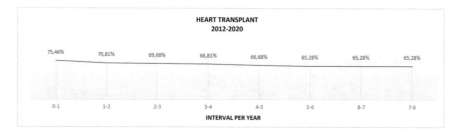

Fig. 4.5 Heart transplant survival scale

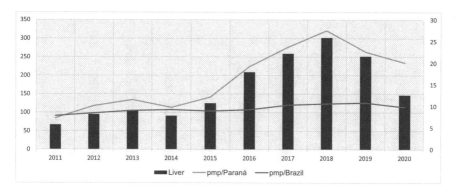

Fig. 4.6 Absolute and proportional liver transplant progress. (*pmp* per million population)

Liver Transplant

A total of 1653 liver transplants were performed, of which chronic hepatitis B and C, alcoholism, and primary liver cancer were the most common indication that arose.

The procedure has maintained absolute and proportional numbers above the national average (Fig. 4.6) and is currently performed in nine centers.

In 1 year, liver transplant's survival reaches 77.30% and, in 5 years, 72.14% (Fig. 4.7).

Kidney Transplantation

A total of 3525 kidney transplants were performed, with the most frequent etiologies being multifactorial chronic kidney disease, hypertensive disease, and diabetes.

Kidney transplantation is the most common procedure performed in the country, and proportionally to the population, Paraná ranked behind the national average early in the decade. Only from 2015 onward, the state has exceeded the national average and since then has remained above it – due to a large amount of lost ground

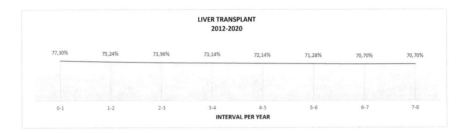

Fig. 4.7 Liver transplant survival scale

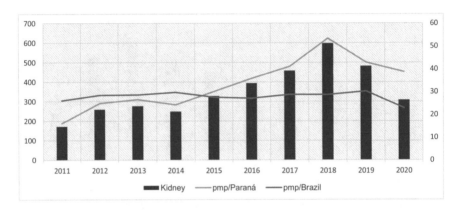

Fig. 4.8 Absolute and proportional kidney transplant progress. (*pmp* per million population)

to recover (Fig. 4.8). Currently, kidney transplantation is performed in 15 transplant centers.

The increase of kidney transplant numbers from deceased donors has a positive side effect. A kidney transplant from a living donor – 1362 performed in this period – is losing its power as the primary therapeutic route for patients with chronic kidney disease who need renal replacement therapy (Fig. 4.9).

As the availability of organs from deceased donors increases, the strain over the living donor system decreases. Living donor kidney transplants have their qualities, effectiveness, and safety well established in the literature (Manfro et al., 2014), yet living donation cannot be used as a crutch for an inefficient deceased donor organ procurement system.

In relative terms, living donor transplant has increased and is expected to stabilize at a range of 5–10 transplants/pmp per year (ABTO, 2019).

Kidney transplantation has an 84.74% one-year survival rate and a 76.19% five-year survival rate. It is worth pointing out that despite its impact on life expectancy, this transplant procedure has its most significant effect on receivers' life quality (Evans et al., 1985), which is not measured by the survival scale (Fig. 4.10).

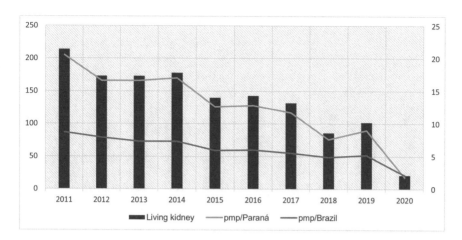

Fig. 4.9 Absolute and proportional kidney living donor transplant progress. (*pmp* per million population)

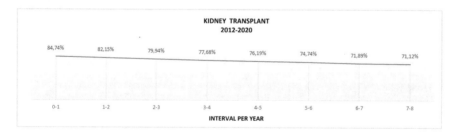

Fig. 4.10 Kidney transplant survival scale

Pancreas Transplant

A number of 213 pancreas transplants were performed, 180 simultaneous pancreas-kidney transplant procedures, and 33 pancreas-only procedures (Fig. 4.11). The transplant is indicated for type 1 diabetes mellitus patients; being a restricted transplant, it's recommended for severe diseases (Noronha et al., 2011). It is currently performed in three transplant centers.

Double transplantation has a 77.05% one-year survival rate and a 72.52% five-year survival rate; the pancreas alone has a one-year and five-year survival rate of 65.64% and 48.45%, respectively (Figs. 4.12 and 4.13).

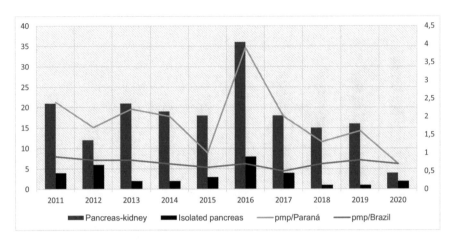

Fig. 4.11 Absolute and proportional pancreas transplant progress. (*pmp* per million population)

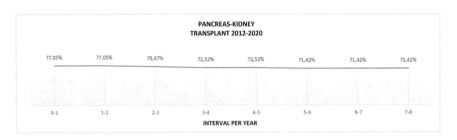

Fig. 4.12 Pancreas-kidney transplant survival curve

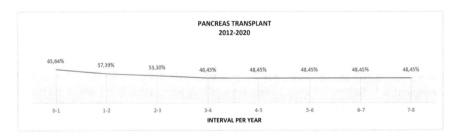

Fig. 4.13 Pancreas transplant survival curve

Corneal Transplant

A total of 8694 corneal transplants, having keratoconus as the main etiology, were performed in the period.

This tissue transplant modality has a well-balanced waiting list, as the supply of tissues meets the demand and remains above the national average (Fig. 4.14). It is currently performed in 29 transplant centers.

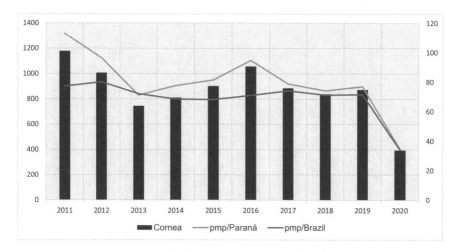

Fig. 4.14 Absolute and proportional progress of corneal transplantation. (*pmp* per million population)

Bone Marrow Transplant

A number of 2711 marrow transplants were performed, being the majority (46%) autologous type, (32%) halogens related, and (22%) unrelated halogens (Fig. 4.15). Nine transplant centers perform autologous marrow transplantation, halogen related in five transplant centers, and unrelated in four transplant centers.

Posttransplant Sector

The initial approach of reorganizing the processes of active search and transplantation access gradually revealed the need to improve posttransplant processes as a natural consequence of the system's growth and the number of transplants performed.

This sector has the prerogative of the follow-up transplants performed in the state and involves several items such as surveillance transmission of bacterial, viral, and fungal infections; donor's culture monitoring; handling of adverse events reported by the transplant teams; and acting as a communication channel among several transplant centers that eventually received the organs from a specific donor involved in an adverse event. These are not random or accidental events, as transplants, whether of organs, tissues, or cells, are not risk-free, and it is imperative to have this sort of quality control.

The enhancements of all stages of the donation-transplant process resulted in the pursuit of improvement, acknowledgment of weak points, and exaltation of strong points associated with patients' posttransplant survival, including by seeking to bring in expert committees to discuss the topic, in the scope of each organ's State Technical Chambers.

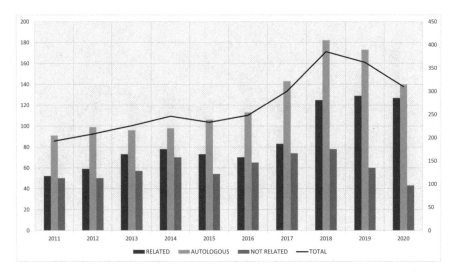

Fig. 4.15 Bone marrow transplant's absolute progress

These debates encouraged the organization of the Paraná Liver and Kidney Transplant Quality Congress, held in 2018, which sought to discuss aspects related to result from improvements, such as donor support, immunogenic issues, and transplant recommendations.

References

ABTO. (2019). In V. D. Garcia (Ed.), *RBT - Registro Brasileiro de Transplantes*. ABTO - Associação Brasileira de Transplante de Órgãos.
ABTO. (2020). In V. D. Garcia (Ed.), *RBT - Registro Brasileiro de Transplantes*. ABTO - Associação Brasileira de Transplante de Órgãos.
BRASIL. (2017). *Portaria de Consolidação n°4, de 28 de setembro de 2017*. Ministério da Saúde.
Evans, R. W., Manninen, D. L., Jr Garrison, L. P., Hart, L. G., Blagg, C. R., Gutman, R. A., Hull, A. R., & Lowrie, E. G. (1985). The quality of life of patients with end-stage renal disease. *The New England Journal of Medicine, 312*, 553–559.
Instituto Nacional do Câncer, I. (2021). *Atlas on-line de mortalidade*. Ministério da Saúde.
Manfro, R. C., Noronha, I. L., & Filho, A. P. E. S. (2014). *Manual de Transplante Renal*. Barueri SP.
Manzei, A. (2016). Organ shortage as a structural problem in transplantation medicine. In R. J. Jox, G. Assadi, & G. Marckmann (Eds.), *Organ transplantation in times of donor shortage*. Springer International Publishing.
Noronha, I. L., Gonzalez, A. M., & Ferreira, R. (2011). *Manual de Transplante de Pâncreas*. Segmento Farma Editores.
Paraná, G. D. E. D. (2018). In S. E. D. Transplantes (Ed.), *Plano Estadual de Doação e Transplantes de Órgãos e Tecidos 2018–2022*.

Chapter 5
Interference of the Human Factor in the Efficiency of Paraná's Transplant System

The Maturity of the System

A transplant system develops when the standard operating procedures are established when data is no longer random and becomes consistent and especially when the population comes to believe in the system.

An actual donor is the outcome of an equation of an identified potential donor, diagnosed, properly cared for, and family consent granted. The more identification and diagnostic confirmation, with less refusal, the greater will be the availability of organs for transplantation.

In Paraná State, over the last decade, we have observed a constant increase of potential donors' detection and actual donation, though any growth must be linked to some reference.

Let's start our comparison concerning Brazil. Regarding potential donors, proportionally to the population, the state began to move away in 2012, ending 2020 with a 100% higher rate (Fig. 5.1).

Regarding actual donors, the state reached 47.7 pmp (2018), 43.8 pmp (2019), and 41.5 pmp (2020), ending up with a rate 162% higher than the national average (Fig. 5.2).

Concerning Latin America, considering the year 2019 to exclude the hassle of the pandemic year, Uruguay is the country with the best effective donor rates, with 20.4 pmp. This is followed by Brazil (17), Argentina (13.3), Cuba (12.4), Chile (10), Colombia (8.9), Peru (7.5), and Mexico (4.5) (ABTO, 2019). All Paraná manages to present higher numbers.

Moving on to North America, the United States (33.3) and Canada (21.9) begin to show better numbers. In Europe, the competition is more intense; Spain (49.9) and Croatia (41.2) are true record holders and role models for our state. The countries that follow in the European *ranking* – Portugal and Belgium – with 33.6 effective donors/pmp are already below Paraná's rates. It's worth stressing that European

F. Silveira, A. T. C. G. Badoch, *Effective Public Health Policy in Organ Donation*, SpringerBriefs in Public Health, https://doi.org/10.1007/978-3-030-99288-0_5

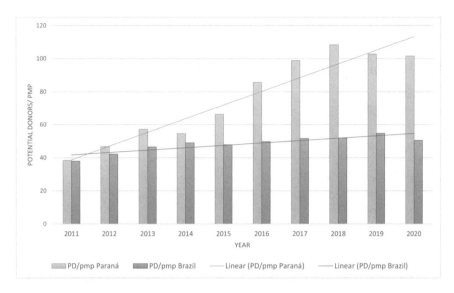

Fig. 5.1 Brazil-Paraná potential donors per million population comparatives. (*pmp* per million population)

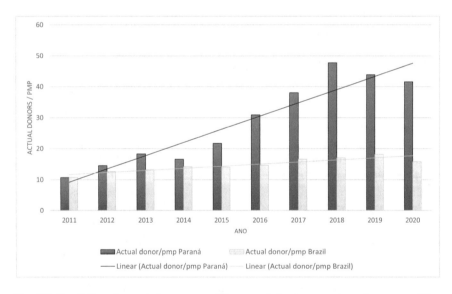

Fig. 5.2 Brazil-Paraná actual donors per million population comparatives. (*pmp* per million population)

countries include organ donors under the circulatory arrest category in their estimates, a condition not foreseen in the Brazilian legislation.

At last, it is necessary to compare it with the Spanish system, known as the world's best identification and capture organ system. Many regions of the world used its standard as a *benchmark*, often referred to as the "Spanish miracle." Its quality audit metrics and productivity goals indicate that 2.2% of people who die in hospitals are potential donors (Matesanz et al., 2017).

Upon analyzing this ratio in terms of hospital deaths in Paraná State, we created the Paraná Index (PI). As per analysis, the Paraná Index was lower than one that did not achieve the recommended goal set by the Spanish system, and higher than one, the goal was surpassed.

Paraná's system analysis under the perspective of the Paraná Index shows that year over year (2011–2019), there was an average increase in the index in the health regions that comprise the OPOs (Fig. 5.3).

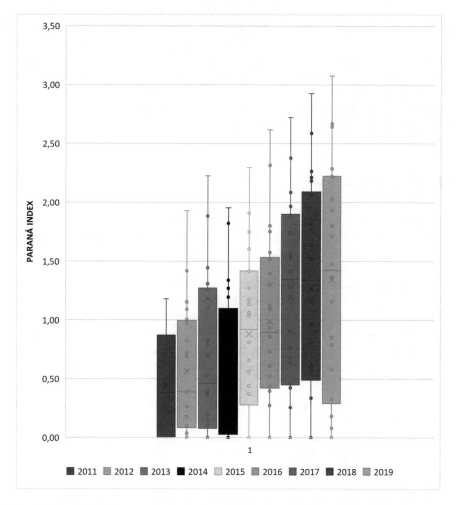

Fig. 5.3 Paraná Index average in the state's regional health departments. (The PI average is displayed by the X, boxes, and the standard variation and circles the positions of the health regional offices)

In 2016, the Paraná Index average of all regional health areas got close to the target rate (0.99 ± 0.73). In 2019, thirteen health regions – 59% of the total – had PI$\geq$1. The PI has steadily grown annually statewide, achieved an average of 1.34 in 2019 or 34% more than the Spanish target.

The highest Paraná Index was achieved in 2019 by 15 RS – Maringá, with 3.08, which means that the region exceeded by three times the potential donor's identification goal recommended by the standard Spanish pattern. The OPO in which 100% of the health regions met or exceeded the goal was the Cascavel OPO.

Paraná State Transplant System model is able to meet and surpass the Spanish pattern target to identify potential organ donors. Although it is an operational reference, it must be reminded that the Spanish pattern is not reproduced in the same format in Paraná State. The combined in-hospital performance of the CIHDOTTS, with the state role, the OPOs, constitutes a hybridization of the Spanish model.

However, the journey is not over as identifying potential donors is the chain's first step, which leads to the donation, followed by the family approach and consent to transform the potential donor into an actual donor. This change is a multidimensional process, influenced by economic aspects, healthcare access, hospital organization, the transplant system, and cultural aspects. Will it be possible to identify which of these aspects prevails the most?

National Projection

The restructuring initiation of the State Transplant System began in 2011, and its first results became apparent in 2012, as the state started to outperform the Brazilian average of effective donors/pmp. The healthy competition between the best socioeconomic development states in the country was fierce.

Its biggest opponent – Santa Catarina – was highlighted in the editorials of the Brazilian Transplant Registry (RBT), the Brazilian Association of Organ Transplantation (ABTO) channel, and the most relevant report of the Brazilian transplant system. In 2011, the RBT brought the following:

> …While Brazil reached nearly 11 donors per million inhabitants, Santa Catarina state reached 25 effective donors per million inhabitants, the best result ever reached by a Brazilian state…. (ABTO, 2011)

Santa Catarina's leadership continued to stand out in 2015, when Paraná totaled 21.7 actual donors/pmp:

> …Santa Catarina, like in the last ten years, remains outstanding when it comes to donations (30.2 pmp)…. (ABTO, 2015)

In 2016, there is the first reference of Paraná in the RBT editorial:

> …The leading states in terms of demand were: SC (36.8 pmp), due to its similar rate when compared to the best-performing countries of the world, and PR (30.9 pmp), due to its fast growth of 42% this year…. (ABTO, 2016)

In 2017, both neighbors started to gap with the remaining states of the federation:

> …SC (40.8 pmp) stood out with a 10.9% increase and PR (38.0 pmp) with a 26.2% increase, the only states that exceeded 30 pmp donors…. (ABTO, 2017)

In 2018, Paraná surpassed Santa Catarina for the first time:

> …With extraordinary donation rates over 40 pmp, PR (47.7 pmp) and SC (41.0 pmp) stood out, and PR also had a potential donor report rate of 108 pmp, even higher than the maximum expected (100 pmp)…. (ABTO, 2018)

The dispute remained tight and was always faced as encouraging with each Brazilian Association of Organ Transplantation report; in 2019, it reported the following:

> …They stood out with potential donors notification rates over >100 pmp , DF (106.6) and PR (102.7); with effective donor rates over 40 pmp, SC (47.2) and PR (43.8); with donation effectiveness rate over 50%, SC (54%) and with family authorization rates over 70%, SC (75%), PR (74%) and RJ (71%)…. (ABTO, 2019)

To conclude, in 2020, we had the pandemic year, whose editorial brought the following:

> …The merit of PR and SC must be recognized, although with a slight drop (13% and 19%), they kept a high rate of actual donors (41.5 and 39.5 pmp), far apart from the other states…. (ABTO, 2020)

Make a Difference

Previously, we saw that the Paraná State Transplant System's evolution settled potential donor's identification numbers, which are comparable or greater than the best metrics. The OPOs gather health regions under their responsibility, trying to integrate or make CIHDOTTs be active in identifying and converting potential donors. **The system takes place in this interaction**.

Paraná State surpasses the Spanish benchmark under the grouped metrics of the OPOs. However, the health regional office's performance is not uniform when analyzed separately. While some exceed it more than two times, 45.4% do not meet the Paraná Index target (Fig. 5.4).

One must suppose that socioeconomic differences may be responsible for the disparity, as the system is tightly linked to the unified health system, which mirrors social inequalities. It is possible to measure these differences through the use of the Municipal Human Development Index (IDHM).

The IDHM is a methodology adjustment of the Human Development Index. It was created and is used by the United Nations (UN) to rank the degree of economic development and life quality of countries. The index brings together three requirements, the opportunity to have a long and healthy life, health; access to knowledge, education; and to enjoy a dignified living standard, income. The purpose of the methodological adjustment development was to adapt the index to the Brazilian cities, states, and regions' development reality, that is, a national context adjustment.

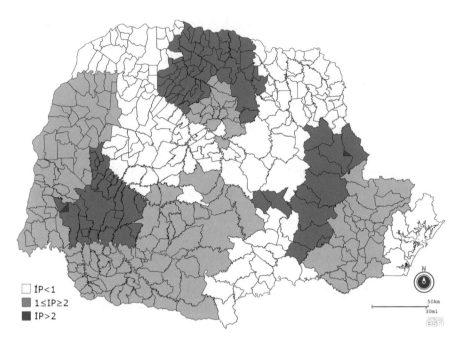

Fig. 5.4 Paraná Index quantitative topic map

Its calculation is composed of more than 200 socioeconomic indicators that expand the understanding of municipal development.

In Paraná, municipalities with high and very high IDHM are responsible for 97.46% of donations, with a significant difference in actual donor rates across the IDHM ranges (low, medium, high, and very high) (Badoch, Silveira, Silveira, et al., 2021).

When applied to the IDHM average of cities that are part of the state's regional health areas, compared to the actual donor's rate, a significant positive linear correction among the indicators is observed, meaning that the higher the IDHM, the higher the actual donor's rates.

Both the scatter graph analysis (Fig. 5.5) and the themed map by health regionals (Fig. 5.6) reveal different donation rates in similar IDHM areas.

And what would be the reasons regions culturally, socially, and economically similar would display such discrepant proportional rates of actual donors?

Reasons for this difference might be connected to the offer of hospital beds, medical specialties, and eventually even interregional transfer agreements for patients with central nervous system diseases. However, this doesn't seem to be an actual cause of influence in the state, as there is no difference in the number of beds available (Table 5.1), and the analysis of hospital deaths, of potential donor's metric basis, doesn't show that the regional health areas with the Paraná Index<1 have fewer deaths than its best-performing counterparts. This data is a reinforcement to argue against the hypothesis of poor access to hospital care.

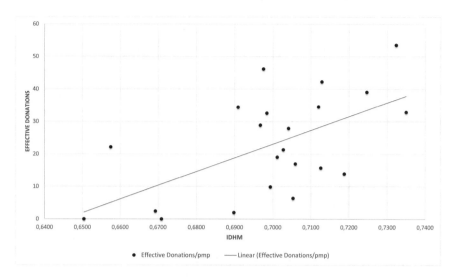

Fig. 5.5 IDHM dispersion diagram of health regionals according to the rate of effective donors/pmp

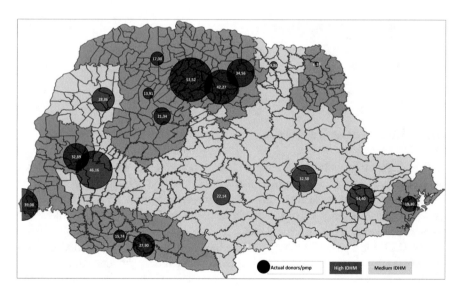

Fig. 5.6 Health regional offices' themed map according to IDHM and actual donations/pmp

The discrepancy observed among similar IDHM ranges presenting different effective donation rates is repeated once this analysis is nationalized. The number of effective donations/pmp grows 418% in the transition from the average to high IDHM range and 129% upon transitioning from high to very high IDHM across Brazilian states (Fig. 5.7).

Table 5.1 Health regional's characteristics according Paraná Index

	IP ≥ 1	IP < 1	p
Health regionals	54.55% ($n = 12$)	45.45% ($n = 10$)	
Paraná index	1.85 ± 0.45	0.40 ± 0.32	0.000[b]
Beds available/population[a]	29.24 ± 0.38	23.02 ± 0.76	0.59
Hospital deaths/population[a]	2.85 ± 0.49	3.31 ± 0.48	0.03[b]

[a]Average in the period (2016–2019); [b]1000

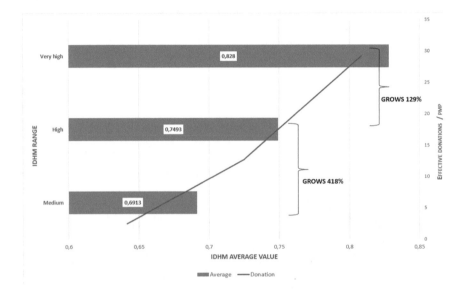

Fig. 5.7 Effective growth of donation/pmp rates according to Brazilian states' IDHM range

It is interesting to observe a positive linear correlation in the high IDHM states but a negative in states with average and very high IDHM (Fig. 5.8).

The dispersion of these data within the average, high, and very high IDHM subgroups reveals a significant difference in actual donor/pmp rates among the states (Badoch, Silveira, Stein, & Giugni, 2021).

The IDHM is a powerful tool to analyze the development of society, and its components – life expectancy, access to health, and education – influence the donation-transplant process: life expectancy, as most donors are stroke victims, most common after the age of 50; access to health because the effective donation results from structured medical care (there is a correlation between the IDHM and the installed health infrastructure); and education because the cultural development level impacts the organ donation refusal rates.

The evidence that is repeated both in the analyses across the state's health regional units and nationwide shows that effective donations are driven by the society's development – assessed by the IHDM. However, this is not the determining

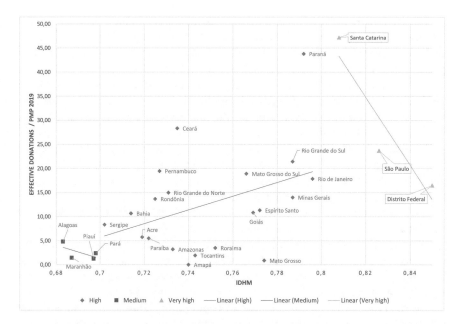

Fig. 5.8 IDHMI dispersion and linear correlation with effective donations/pmp by Brazilian states

feature that distinguishes the performance of the most different organ retrieval systems for transplantation within the same socioeconomic development range.

The resulting equation for donor convertibility depends on quantitative (hospital deaths) and qualitative (access to healthcare and epidemiological profile of the population) variables. Analyzing these two indicators, in terms of hospital death ratios (Paraná Index) and Municipal Human Development Index (IDHM), shows that these indicators indeed influence the conversion rates. Although they do not fully explain the process, regions with similar PI and IDHM have discrepant actual donor rates.

The difference in this equation is people's work. It is the people who make the difference in building an efficient system, shown in the OPO-CIHDOTT interaction.

Move Out of Your Comfort Zone

In the collective health field, the assessment of health programs and services is grounded in pragmatism, a school characterized by the perspective of action rather than contemplation, the science's need to strive for a social outcome.

The medical and public health background of the State Transplant System's coordination established regular evaluation processes, represented by the need to submit status reports several times a day, together with remote meetings.

This pragmatic approach was the first paradigm shift because these evaluation processes are rarely included in the executive level, even though health programs – such as the State Transplant System – are nothing more than a state's or country's public policy translation (Furtado, 2012).

This continuous interaction of the State Transplant Center coordination with the OPOs, heavily influenced by the general coordination profile, was eased by technology arrival, which allowed real-time interaction, assisted by uninterrupted use of voice and video interaction mechanisms.

The state character of the OPOs managed to energize a command chain notion that encouraged and enforced the OPOs' interaction with the CIHDOTTS, stimulating local solution development and strengthening the SUS's decentralized nature, characterizing the second paradigm breach.

The constant interaction – general coordination, OPOs, CIHDOTTs – definitely constituted the keystone of Paraná State Transplant System's success, which managed to imprint efficiency, efficacy, and effectiveness on the unified health system. As previously demonstrated, this triad was set up under similar socioeconomic development conditions, remaining the crucial importance of the careful and relevant actions of the human resources that interacted in this system.

The rhetorical expression – **move out of your comfort zone** – nicely sums up the two paradigm breaches, which are crucial for the system's success, summarized in the general coordinator and agents' actions who interacted in the OPOs and CIHDOTTs throughout Paraná State.

Epilogue

The work built over the decade reported in this piece was a history of love and dedication. The achieved record marks do not represent the perfection of our system; they represent the building of a magnificent system based on the actions of people who managed to make a difference. The framework described in this work is adaptable and can be improved in countries that lack socioeconomic development indexes as strong as those in Europe or Anglo-Saxon countries.

The process was not the action of a single person, but rather of public staff from the State Transplant Center and Organ Procurement Organizations, working as an actual team, a team that effectively responded to daily demands. Under no circumstances OPOs should step out of the hospitals, interacting with the professionals of the Intra-Hospital Committee on Organ and Tissue Donation for Transplants and critical care areas, always aiming to improve the process. Our acknowledgment and appreciation for the dedication of the valuable members of the Intra-Hospital Committee on Organ and Tissue Donation for Transplants and to all the professionals who work with critically ill patients in Paraná. They are the foundation of the whole structure, as they are the ones who first identify potential donors and initiate the process. Therefore, when analyzing the data of all these years, it is possible to observe the work progression and development with all the characteristics, qualities, and difficulties of our OPOs.

The data analysis enables us to claim that if we operate under the best of performances, a rate of 69 effective donors per million population can be achieved. It is a bold goal yet consistent with those who stay out of their comfort zone.

References

ABTO. (2011). In V. D. Garcia (Ed.), *RBT - Registro Brasileiro de Transplantes*. ABTO - Associação Brasileira de Transplante de Órgãos.

ABTO. (2015). In V. D. Garcia (Ed.), *RBT - Registro Brasileiro de Transplantes*. ABTO - Associação Brasileira de Transplante de Órgãos.

ABTO. (2016). In V. D. Garcia (Ed.), *RBT - Registro Brasileiro de Transplantes*. ABTO - Associação Brasileira de Transplante de Órgãos.

ABTO. (2017). In V. D. Garcia (Ed.), *RBT - Registro Brasileiro de Transplantes*. ABTO - Associação Brasileira de Transplante de Órgãos.

ABTO. (2018). In V. D. Garcia (Ed.), *RBT - Registro Brasileiro de Transplantes*. ABTO - Associação Brasileira de Transplante de Órgãos.

ABTO. (2019). In V. D. Garcia (Ed.), *RBT - Registro Brasileiro de Transplantes*. ABTO - Associação Brasileira de Transplante de Órgãos.

ABTO. (2020). In V. D. Garcia (Ed.), *RBT - Registro Brasileiro de Transplantes*. ABTO - Associação Brasileira de Transplante de Órgãos.

Badoch, A. T., Silveira, F., Silveira, F. P., Von Stein, A., & Giugni, J. (2021). Doadores de órgãos efetivos no Paraná e correlação com o Índice de Desenvolvimento Humano Municipal. *Revista de Saúde Pública do Paraná, 4*.

Badoch, A. T. C., Silveira, F., Stein, A. V., & Giugni, J. R. (2021). Taxa de doações efetivas no Brasil e correlação com o Índice de Desenvolvimento Humano Municipal. *JBT - Jornal Brasileiro de Transplantes, 24*, 80.

Furtado, J. P. (2012). Avaliação de Programas e Serviços em Saúde. In G. W. S. Campos (Ed.), *Tratado de Saúde Coletiva. Segunda*. Hucitec.

Matesanz, R., Dominguez-Gil, B., Coll, E., Mahillo, B., & Marazuela, R. (2017). How Spain reached 40 deceased organ donors per million population. *American Journal of Transplantation, 17*, 1447–1454.

Index

Printed in the United States
by Baker & Taylor Publisher Services